"Before I recommend a book, there are three criteria it must meet: First, the author needs to be knowledgable, practical, and "walk their talk." Second, the book needs to be non-judgmental in the approach with zero hype and no false promises. Third, it needs to work! Dr. Willis in *Food is the Cure* achieves all three."

**Dr. Lee Jampolsky,**
Best Selling Author of *"Smile for no Good Reason"*

"This is an easy to read book but also cites the evidence behind Dr. Willis' methods. I think all patients with BMI over 29 should read the book and fly to success!"

**Dr. Andy Skiles**

"This will change your life … It is the most honest and genuine book where the intention is to clearly help people and change the way they think about weight loss."

**Professor Inderjit Kaur, India**

"When you incorporate fun elements that involve friends and family, exercise becomes easy and rewarding. That's why I think the child curls are a great example of thinking outside of the box."

**Dale L. Roberts**
Best Selling Author of over 40 fitness books

This book is dedicated to my loving parents who were truly empowering, especially when I struggled following an "Unsurvivable plane crash"! (See Foreward.)

**Tomorrow's victory ... starts today!**

Special thanks to my mentors, patients, and friends who proved my methods (with pictures) in their Rightsize, weight loss!

ISBN: 9781713448303
ISBN: 9780578577111
ISBN: 9780578577128

# ***Food is the Cure***
*for the Overweight Disease!*



For More Pictures of Recipes and Aerobic-surges exercises go to

**www.DrBuckWillis.com**

# FOREWARD

**My life started again 30 years ago with an "Unsurvivable plane crash"!** After enduring a 3-year series of 16 sequential operations to rebuild my legs, I later squatted a lifetime high of 505 pounds and became passionate about helping others from my experiences. The crash also resulted in a moderate brain injury, and as victory I earned four degrees including my medical degree in the British Commonwealth (MBBS) and PhD in kinesiology.

**However, I was obese when I started med school.** My Body Mass Index (BMI) was 32 and a value over 30 is categorically obese. I was my first patient and dropped 40.lbs. It was still a daily challenge until I later tested to identify the causes of this disease (Hidden food allergies). Now my weight continues to drop, and I'm 55.lbs lighter than in med school!

After also earning my PhD in kinesiology, I directed research in clinical rehabilitation and I was later chosen to be a fellow of the American College of Sports Medicine. My post-doc learning was in holistic medicine and I am blessed to now serve as an integrative, board-certified holistic physician and accredited scientist. Thank you, God!

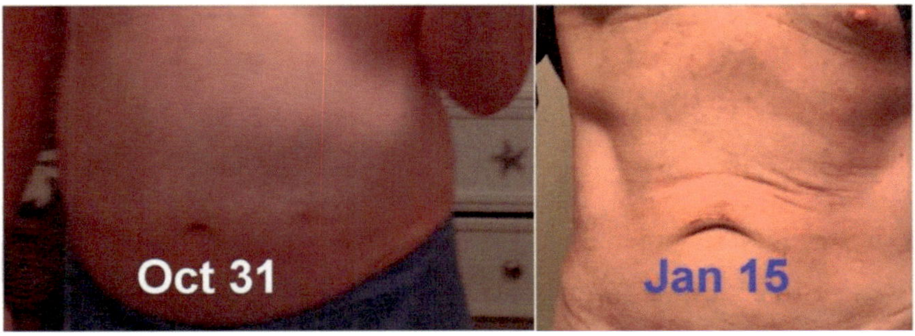


In the last 20 years, the USA, UK, Canada, and Australia have become more obese. We need to use scientifically-proven methods to cure the verweight disease that burdens over 70% of our neighbors.

**Curing the overweight disease starts by determining the causes, which are different for each person.** The most common causes include a combination of food chemicals/preservatives/sweeteners, hidden food allergies, lectin food inflammation, endocrine imbalances, menopause, and other sources of GI inflammation.

Let's start this journey with many *bites of victory* saying, "**Eat More and Exercise Less!**"

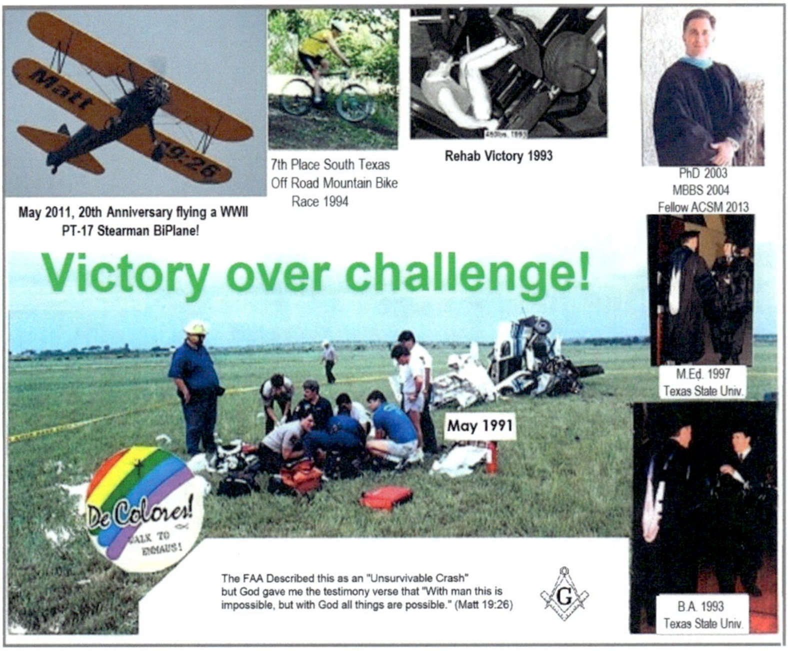
Matt
19:26
May 2011, 20th Anniversary flying a WWII
PT-17 Stearman BiPlane!
7th Place South Texas
Off Road Mountain Bike
Race 1994
Rehab Victory 1993
PhD 2003
MBBS 2004
Fellow ACSM 2013
Victory over challenge!
M.Ed. 1997
Texas State Univ.
May 1991
De Colores!
WALK TO
EMMAUS!
The FAA Described this as an "Unsurvivable Crash"
but God gave me the testimony verse that "With man this is
impossible, but with God all things are possible." (Matt 19:26)
B.A. 1993
Texas State Univ.

# CHAPTER 1
# Eat More and Exercise Less

Each chapter will start with an empathetic taste of victory. You can read my weight loss testimony in the forward.

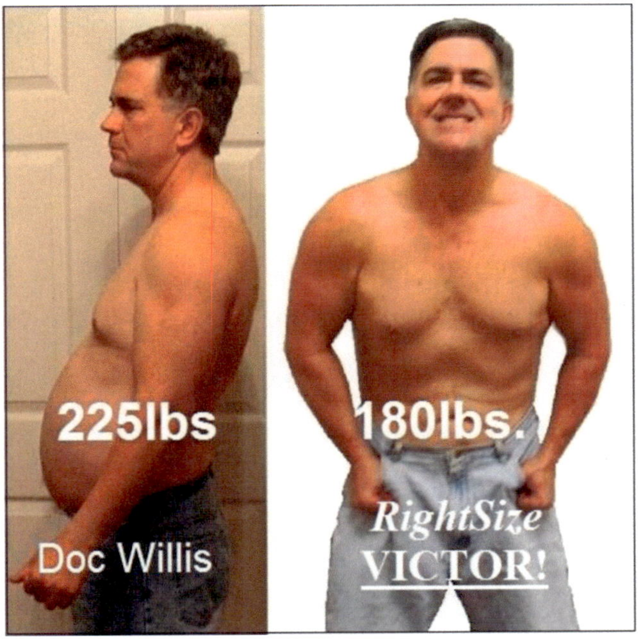


**The first step to losing weight is to stop continually gaining weight!** We will learn methods to identify the causes and use delicious recipes (Eating more) and quick, 2-minute exercises for your victory!

Food is both the cause and the cure of this disease. My patients drop an average of -46 pounds, -30 inches, and -30% body fat by first eliminating the causes of this disease.

Traditional medicine says "a disease is an acquired condition that produces specific signs or symptoms, which can be reduced with controlled treatment." Being overweight or obese IS a disease. It's no one's fault and it is NOT from eating too much, unless it's too much high fructose corn syrup and too much TBHQ chemicals!

When the body has an inflammatory gastral reaction and/or a low-level (subacute) allergic reaction to a food, it lowers our metabolism and puts a body into the "survival mode" that causes us to gain weight. What if this happens to us several times a week or even several times each day? In such a case, how could we not gain weight? Hidden food allergies are estimated to affect 75% of the US population and the majority of people in the UK, Canada, and Australia. The same percentages are also overweight.

Now we need to learn how to use food to raise the metabolism naturally. The secret is to eat the right, natural foods more often (in single portion sizes). Think of fast food's "mega size" as something that causes a "mega waistline" versus the lean bodybuilders (who eat five to six times a day) have low body fat! Here is a quick overview of scientifically proven methods for fat loss and permanent weight loss (after the causes are removed).

**Research has proven that eating smaller, single portion-size meals or snacks (eaten five times per day) increases the metabolism and burns more fat as fuel.** An old study of Olympic boxers proved this (Iwao et al, 1996). All boxers had the same training schedule and they all ate the same exact total quantity and quality (selections) of the same foods. The only variable was the number of times per day each athlete ate from this daily portion of food.

The scientists divided the total mass of food into either two meals or six meals. While all of the boxers lost the same amount of weight before a competition, the 6-meal group lost 75% more fat! Eating five meals or snacks per day will help you lose fat (each meal/snack must be less than two cups per meal).

It has been shown in many new research studies that brief bouts of exercise in the aerobic threshold (heart rate at 75% of calculated maximum) burns more fat and is equivalent to working out for a much longer amount of time. I led a multi-center study in 2016 that showed performing a brief, **aerobic surge exercise** for 2 minutes, 5 times a day, achieved an -18.lbs weight loss with -18 inches in just 60 days without any dietary modifications!

The control group that was simply instructed to "exercise more" actually gained one pound and one inch.

To calculate your aerobic threshold, subtract your age from 220. That is your estimated maximum heart rate (even if you were running away from a lion). Take that number and multiply it by 0.75 to determine your estimated aerobic threshold. (For example, 220 - 50 years old = 170 x 0.75 = 127 beats per minute). I suggest using a quick bicycle ride to increase your heart rate (the bike keeps the weight off your knees). Simply get your heart rate up to the aerobic threshold for two minutes and then leisurely ride back home.

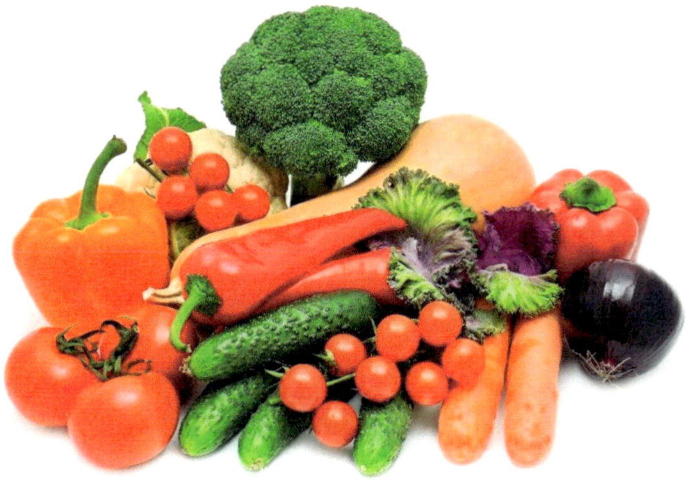

**Eating natural foods** has also been proven beneficial in weight loss. Add a slice of apple or a few blueberries to every portion size meal (within the two-cup maximum). Even the top nutritionist with the National

Institute of Health (NIH) says that natural foods make one "feel satiated" (you feel full and no longer hungry), adding that "natural foods are more nutrient-dense." A study performed by Poulsen et al (2014) examined change in weight and blood pressure after replacing daily processed food products with all natural foods in the New Nordic Diet (NND).

One hundred and eighty-one obese subjects (average BMI > 30) participated in this diet change study. There was no exercise required, but all foods were tracked. In six months, the subjects who ate the NND experienced a significant drop in weight and blood pressure.

How can you combine the frequent eating of natural foods and aerobic surges into your daily schedule? The answer is to plan and forecast your meals with quick exercise bouts for daily victory!

You can use these tools even if you are dining with the President. Don't run around the tables or you might get arrested (or Trump will fire you), but you can precede the dining event by climbing the stairs. Take the stairs and briskly walk up 120 steps. (That is what we do on the cruise ship before each meal.) If you have food selection options, choose the natural or "clean" foods. If you don't have a choice, then only eat the clean foods you are given. Even if your entire meal comes from processed, packaged survival food, eat a slice of apple for dessert.

Start today by measuring your body weight first and circumferences first thing in the morning. (Use the body summation on the last page of this book.) You can also find a clinic to measure your body fat (The 'BodPod' testing chamber can be found in most large cities.). That is needed because your initial changes will be predominantly in fat, which is the lightest substance in the body, so the scales may not change as much as the fat loss.

***Digest This:*** Use the PAN-5 protocols with this 30-day formula to stop this disease from progressing and help you lose fat and weight. Then combine this with elimination of hidden food allergens for a lifetime cure! (Email us and we'll send you a blood test and phlebotomist, FBW@DocWillis.org)

# CHAPTER 2

## Where Are We Now?

**Taste of Victory**: Are you sitting at a desk all day, struggling to "find the time" to exercise or follow a reduction diet? "Kim" had that challenge. First, we completed a nutritional assessment to eliminate the known causes of this disease (i.e. high fructose corn syrup). Then we tested her blood for reactions to 250 foods (even egg whites vs yolks). Her food allergen testing came back with 80 positive (allergy) results. Eliminating food allergies meant the weight flew off!

Her outstanding effort to include natural methods to help raise her metabolism throughout the day. **In her first 2 months, she dropped -25 pounds of pure fat, plus -25 inches (without drugs or diets)!** Kim felt her treatment plan was the "easiest" (that she's tried) but did require mental planning (forecasting her success). Kim had tried several different diets in the past with no lasting success until she used the methods you are reading.

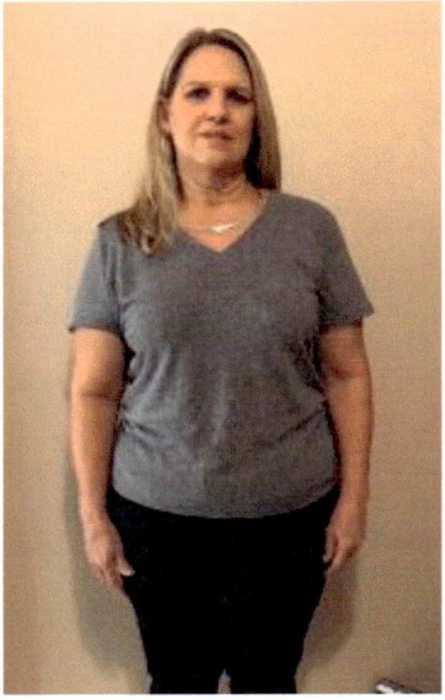

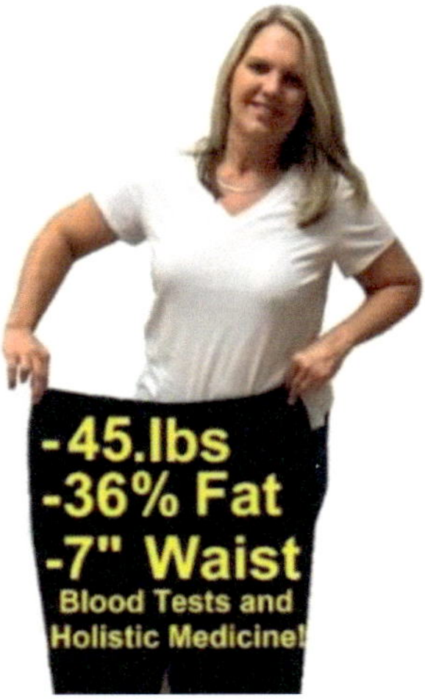


## Known Causes of the Overweight Disease

Our bodies were **not** made to consume the often toxic chemicals included in commercially-produced, packaged food products. Here is a list of the chemicals commonly found in processed foods.

**Arsenic** in grape and apple juice. This is a carcinogenic substance that has been linked to cancer of the lungs, kidney, and bladder. It's been found added to apple juice.

**Aspartame (artificial sweetener)** found in many "diet" sodas. Research has shown that diet sodas actually slow down the metabolism, increase carbohydrate cravings, and lead to weight gain. There are numerous diseases that are caused, enhanced, or aggravated by these chemicals.

Aspartame is carcinogenic and has been clearly associated with brain tumors and lymphoma. Plus it contributes to pathologies such as migraine headaches, diabetes, multiple sclerosis, Parkinson's, Alzheimer's, fibromyalgia, and more. The bottom line is that natural sugar cane, when consumed in small doses, will actually raise your metabolism!

**Bisphenol A (BPA) and phthalates** are found in plastics and bind to food. BPA has been linked to abnormally accelerated pubescent development in children. These can be found in "microwave safe" plastic bowls. Microwave action frees the BPA, which then attaches to food particles. If you use a microwave, transfer the food to a glass dish before heating.

**Camauba wax** in chewing gums, can cause cancer and oral tumors.

**Caramel food coloring (4-Mel)** is found in drinks like Pepsi One and even Pop-Tarts. This additive has been proven to be carcinogenic. In a test completed by *Consumer Reports* (2013), the levels of 4-Mel in Pepsi One and Malta Goya were at levels >29 micrograms, which is higher than the maximum allowed without caution labels in California. These drinks should have a label that reads "possibly carcinogenic to humans," similar to the labels required on cigarettes.

**High fructose corn syrup (HFCS)** is the Enemy in the weight loss battle! It is found in packaged pastries (some commercial breads), salad dressings, cereal, and even canned vegetables. In fact, there are few commercially-processed foods that do not have HFCS. It is actually one of the highest sources sweeteners in commercial food, but these are "wasted calories" because they burn quickly and easily with limited benefit and transition immediately into body fat. HFCS has also been shown to raise LDL, which is the "bad cholesterol." If you eat at a restaurant that does not have a pastry chef, the sweets are probably packaged commercial foods with HFCS. It is also a direct contributing factor in Type II Diabetes!

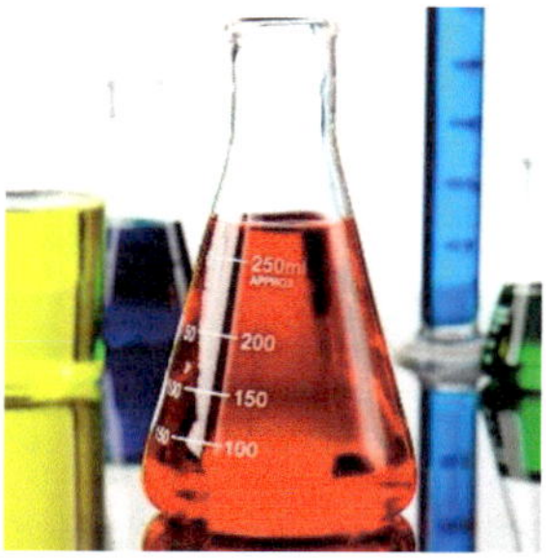

**Monosodium glutamate (MSG)** is used to enhance the flavor in protein-rich foods, like fish, meats, and milk. This is commonly used in commercial, restaurant-prepared foods where you are not able to see the ingredient labels.

MSG can cause migraine headaches, chronic inflammation, liver cancer, central obesity, fatty liver disease and it contributes to decreased insulin sensitivity (Type II Diabetes). Fatty liver disease can also lead to cirrhosis. We think of soup as a healthy food that we feed family members who are ill, but read the labels and MSG is even included in Campbell's minestrone soup.

**Potassium bromate** is found in commercial bread products. This is a substance shown to cause cancer in animal studies and is in several packaged "healthy breads."

**Red and yellow dyes** (Red-40, Tartazine, Azo Dye, and Sunset Yellow) are still in children's macaroni and cheese! These chemicals are banned for foods produced in the UK, Netherlands, and Sweden, however these chemicals are still in American processed foods. During the last 50 years, use of these toxins has increased by 500%. They cause damage to the immune system and errors in cell replication. Some children who have eaten these toxins may develop abnormal chromosome replication patterns. There are even published hypotheses stating that food dyes could be causing increased incidence of ADHD

Whimsical green and yellow cake batter ice cream packed with fabulous purple sugar cookie chips and swirling with ribbons of pinkish frosting.

# Nutrition Facts

**Serving size 2/3 CUP (103g)**

**Amount per serving**

| **Calories** | **270** |
|---|---|
| | **% Daily Value*** |
| **Total Fat** 14g | **18%** |
| Saturated Fat 9g | **45%** |
| *Trans* Fat 0g | |
| **Cholesterol** 30mg | **10%** |
| **Sodium** 65mg | **3%** |
| **Total Carbohydrate** 34g | **12%** |
| Dietary Fiber 0g | **0%** |
| Total Sugars 29g | |
| Includes 23g Added Sugars | **46%** |
| **Protein** 3g | |
| Vitamin D 0mcg | 0% |
| Calcium 132mg | 10% |
| Iron 0mg | 0% |
| Potassium 104mg | 2% |

* The % Daily Value (DV) tells you how much a nutrient in a serving of food contributes to a daily diet. 2,000 calories a day is used for general nutrition advice

**INGREDIENTS:** CREAM, NONFAT MILK, RED ICING (SUGAR, CORN OIL, COCONUT OIL, CORN STARCH, SOY LECITHIN, SOYBEAN OIL, RED 40, SALT, NATURAL FLAVOR), SUGAR, HIGH FRUCTOSE CORN SYRUP, PURPLE COOKIE CHIP (SUGAR, COCONUT OIL, HYDROGENATED COCONUT OIL, CORNSTARCH, SOY LECITHIN, VEGETABLE JUICE [COLOR], NATURAL FLAVOR, BLUE 1 LAKE), CAKE BATTER FLAVOR (WATER, CORN SUGAR, FRUCTOSE, SUGAR, WHEAT FLOUR, BUTTER [CREAM, SALT,], NATURAL AND ARTIFICIAL FLAVORS, NONFAT DRY MILK, SALT, MODIFIED CORN STARCH, YELLOW 5), CORN SYRUP, WHEY, MONO- & DIGLYCERIDES, GUAR GUM, POLYSORBATE 80, CARRAGEENAN, BLUE 1, YELLOW 5, YELLOW 6, RED 40.

**CONTAINS: MILK, SOY, WHEAT.**

**Refined vegetable oils** are found in foods ranging from animal crackers to chocolate-covered peanuts. These include soybean oil, safflower oil, canola oil, and peanut oil. These products can cause headaches and digestive disorders, and are linked to heart disease and cancer. Such oils are common in packaged snack foods. (Canola beans were modified to be resistant to the Round Up weed killer. When they spray canola beans with such chemicals, who eventually consumes it?)

**Sodium benzoate** is in salad dressing and carbonated beverages. This preservative is a known carcinogen and may damage DNA, which would result in damaged cell structures from the point on consumption on.

**Sodium nitrate or nitrite** can be found in lunch eat, hotdogs, corned beef, smoked fish, etc. Our bodies were not made to deal with ingesting such artificial lab hemicals. In response to these chemicals, our bodies start producing excessive, useless cells, which can eventually become a tumor. These chemicals have been shown to cause cancer in the liver and pancreas. The United States Food and Drug Administration (FDA) tried to ban use of sodium nitrite in the 1970s, but political lobbyists controlled the politicians, who stopped funding of this investigation.

**Sodium phosphate** is found in cheeses, salad dressings, packaged snack or breakfast foods, and non-dairy creamers. It has been shown to cause serious kidney damage in some people, including permanent renal damage requiring dialysis. This chemical also causes headaches.

**Sodium sulfite** is common in snack foods such as Chex Mix, some raisins, red wines, and balsamic vinegar. Many people are sensitive to sulfites, which could make this additive an immediately life-threatening toxin. It can also cause celiac disease.

**Sucralose (Splenda®)** is a sweetener in milk, light yogurt, low-fat coffee creamer, cereal bars, light ice cream, licorice, popsicles, canned fruit, factory-baked goods (muffins), light tea, light maple syrup, jams, and jellies. Splenda has also been shown to slow one's metabolism and like other artificial sweeteners, this chemical has been shown to cause leukemia in mice that were exposed to it from before birth. Further studies have shown that sucralose causes DNA damage and cancer in mice. Sucralose is contained in packaged sweets and many dairy products.

**Sulfur dioxide** is found in beer, soft drinks, dried fruit, juices, cordials, wine, vinegar, and potato products. This is a toxic substance prohibited by the FDA in raw fruits and vegetables because it causes bronchial disease and accelerated adverse reactions for people suffering from asthma, hypotension (low blood pressure), emphysema, or cardiovascular disease.

**Tertiary butylhydroquinone (TBHQ)** can be found in some flour-based, packaged food such as Pop-Tarts and breakfast muffins. This is a common food additive/preservative that seems innocent, but consuming just over one gram can cause delirium, nausea, tinnitus (ringing in the ears), and vomiting. It has also been suggested that it contributes to ADHD in children. It may be responsible for affecting estrogen levels in women and research has shown that TBHQ may drop one's metabolism for days at a time.

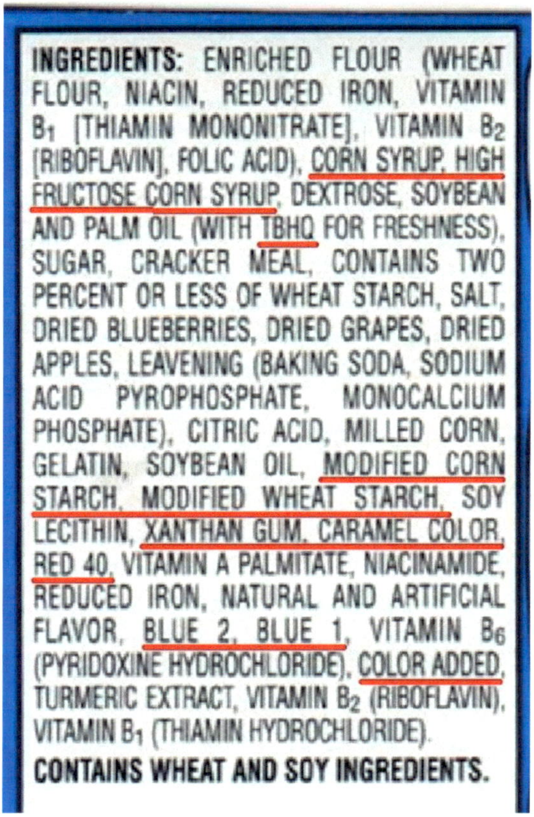


Let's look at a specific example of blueberry Pop-Tarts, which kids love to eat. In reading this expanded label, one can see 15 chemical additives that have been shown to cause or contribute to illness, disease, and cancer. The chemicals are indigestible and contribute to the overweight epidemic. Such synthetic foods do not have the ability to raise the metabolism like natural foods do. How many obese children did we have in 1900?

**A good rule of thumb** is that if a food product has more than five ingredients, you need to examine the label more closely or choose another product. The bottom line should be that if you cannot hold a substance in your hand (i.e. TBHQ), it should not be eaten!

## Inflammatory Foods

Synthetic foods are often the cause of inflammatory reactions. Food additives should be avoided as well. Let's cook like we're back in the 1800s, avoiding these foods:

- Splenda
- High Fructose Corn Syrup
- Sucralose
- Tertiary Butylhydroquinone (TBHQ) in packaged pastries like Pop-Tarts
- Sugar (the worst inflammatory food), though honey and stevia are fine.
- Alcohol, which has been shown to reduce the body's ability to burn fat! Try abstaining from alcohol for 90 days.

Alcohol disrupts the ideal metabolism because it accelerates progression of alcohol to the liver for detoxification.

If I handed you some tertiary butylhydroquinone (TBHQ), what would you do with it? Your body does not know what to do with this chemical either, and it is the preservative that is in almost all packaged carbohydrate food products. It's even in kids' Pop-Tarts! When one digests such a food, the body sees it as a toxin and immediately drops the metabolism because every bit of extra energy is working to expel these toxins!

We have an overweight epidemic caused by excessive, chemical additives in packaged, processed foods. How many chemicals are you eating today? Most commercial food products include chemicals. The bottom line is: why is it good for you to eat something you have never seen being grown in fields?

A famous nutritionist once said, "Eat only things that come from the earth!" Even an "all natural" product of nuts and fruits, listed below, includes sulfur dioxides and other preservatives (Read the ingredients instead of trusting cover labels.).

## Lectins

These are foods with natural pesticides that also cause inflammatory reactions. Have you ever grown tomatoes and noticed that the bugs devour the green leaves, but leave the tomato fruit alone? That is because tomato skins have lectin, a natural insecticide, in the skin of many foods. This will often cause an inflammatory reactions, which again will throw your metabolism to the floor.

Here is a list of some lectin foods:

- Tomato skins (salsa)
- Beans (i.e. pinto and soy)
- Peanuts
- Cashews
- Whole grains (the husk has lectins)
- Barley
- Rice
- Wheat germ
- Zucchini
- Carrots (skin)
- Rhubarb
- Beets
- Mushrooms
- Asparagus
- Turnips
- Cucumbers (skin)
- Pumpkin
- Sweet peppers
- Radishes

***Digest this:*** What were our bodies made to consume? Did your Grandmother also say "We are what we eat?" Did you realize that Adam lived to be 930 years old and **now you <u>can</u> eat the apples** (for better GI motility?)

# CHAPTER 3:
# Why Restrictive Diets Eventually Fail

**Taste of Victory**: "Mary" lost enough body fat to fill a Cheetos bag! She started with a body mass index of 31 (categorically obese) and symptoms of swollen ankles, insomnia, chronic knee pain, and osteoporosis. We removed her food allergens and Mary increased the number of times she was eating meals or snacks (from 2 to 5 per day).

She dropped -12% of her body fat and 13 inches in her first month. After 6 months, she had dropped -35 pounds, -30% body fat, and -34 inches without drugs, diets, or surgery. She said, "It was easy! No food points, calorie counting, or buying packaged foods; I ate natural" (natural foods and more food overall). She's kept her "Rightsize" for a year now!

!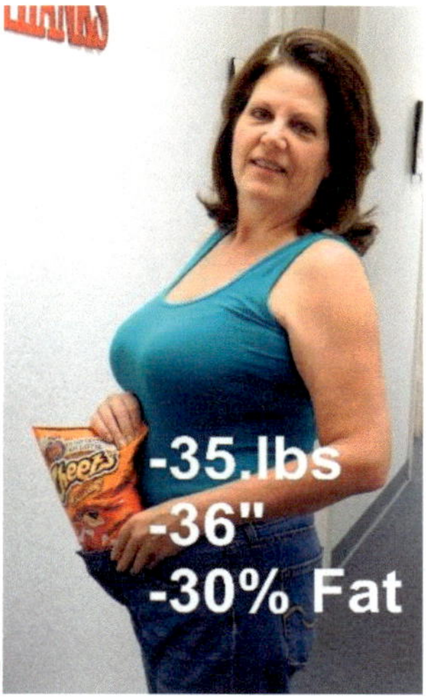

**Diets and other weight loss plans often fail because they don't consciously work to identify and reverse the causes of the overweight disease.** At best, they only treat the symptoms. Fad diets and new, aggressive exercise programs will "shock" the body into quick change, but the body adapts with more "storage" for the next "surprise!" Lifetime weight loss takes more than that shock to regain or obtain one's Rightsize; it takes conscious efforts to identify the causes and eliminate them while also raising the metabolism.

**Metabolic depression** can be an umbrella term for the symptoms of this disease. Whether the cause is simply attributed to processed food choices and inactivity, or more complex causes from hidden food allergies, they all cause an inflammatory reaction which sends metabolism to the floor! We must first determine the cause of obesity to then create a lifetime solution or cure. Let's close the umbrella and stand in the sun!

**Food allergen testing** is an exciting new tool to identify the causes of the overweight disease. This is what has empowered my patients' success for up to 10 years! When the immune system reacts it sends the metabolism to the floor while the body focuses on "detoxifying" the food allergen. You may not be having itching, hives or an upset stomach, but it causes an inflammatory reaction that is a silent cause of the overweight disease.

The good news is that you can have blood testing done anywhere there is a nurse or phlebotomist and FedEx. I've treated patients from the Philippines to the UK from my office in Galveston Texas.

What about research on diet drinks? Numerous studies from Egyptian universities to the Massachusetts General Hospital have shown that drinking diet sodas (with aspartame or sucralose) actually made patients gain weight in comparison to water. Another study also showed that consuming aspartame made people gain more weight, than sugar did. Did you grab that? **Aspartame makes a person gain more weight than Sugar!**

**Counting calories** or food points may work for a while, but again it does not reverse the cause of obesity (Research on "cutting calories" has shown that it actually lowers one's metabolism.). What if you're counting calories in fast food? That is why such programs have limited permanent success in changing the body's shape for a lifetime. How effective are counting calories when one dines with the President or Prime Minister? What variability does the Akins diet offer for Christmas or birthday parties? Instead of counting to eat less, **Eat more natural Food!**

Some weight loss programs work because they combine education, food products, and peer support. These programs have been around for decades, yet our planet has a growing obesity epidemic. This could be due to the lack of focus on reversing the causes of one's disease.

**I say, "Eat cake and lose weight!"** As long as you're not allergic to eggs, wheat, milk, etc. Obviously this does not have the nutrient quality for eating everyday but when we go on a cruise we have one dessert as a separate meal! (Their fresh made desserts are close to 2 cups.) With this program, you will accelerate your metabolism in any circumstance. So test to find the causes of your disease and eat more Earth Foods!

Read the Labels, snd did you notice the page numbers just changed? Read, tand examine,!

***Digest this:*** The old school advice to "eat less and exercise more" is actually the opposite of what science has now shown is needed. Before the sun can rise on your weight loss victory, you first need to remove the causes of this disease! Can you be cured from a chronic respiratory infection without first knowing the exact cause?

# CHAPTER 4
# Hidden Causes of the Disease

**Taste of Victory**: "Rita" wanted a new figure for the last time! She was a busy executive who had tried many diets and did not have time to spend hours at the gym. She came to see me after hearing of a friend's success. I completed a nutritional assessment (including lectin food identification) with a food allergy test that showed significant reactions to 18 common foods (of the 237 tested). She eliminated the food allergens and started the PAN-5 formula. **P** is for a single **Portion size** that can be eaten comfortably within two minutes (<2 cups); **A** is for the 2-minute **Aerobic surge** exercise bout at 75% of max heart rate; **N** is for the **Natural foods** she ate five times a day.

She was not obese but her results were solid. In just her first 10 days, she dropped 6 pounds and 2% of her body fat! There were further challenges, but once she had mastered Rightsize formula, she could always overcome any small setbacks!

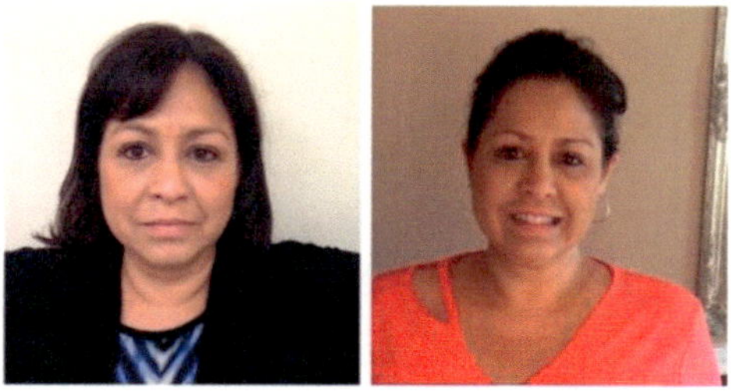

**40-Days: -14**lbs, **-14"**, **-15% Body Fat!**

**Right now, it is estimated that up to 75% of the people in the USA, UK, Canada, and Australia have hidden (subacute) food allergies and rover 70% are overweight.** (The USA has the highest percentage.) Allergic reactions to foods cause inflammatory reactions and such reactions cause weight gain. Let's look deeper into Food allergy testing and elimination. For decades food allergen testing has been used for reduction of migraine headaches and irritable bowel syndrome (IBS). Research has just begun to show that the similar inflammatory reactions that trigger IBS also contribute to the obesity disease.

**White blood cells** have five immunoglobulins (Ig), all of which react differently. The (igE) has the fastest reaction where IgG, IgA, and IgM have slower reactions. Think of IgE as a Flame thrower and IgM as sandpaper. They both yield inflammation but in different ways.

One study by Lewis et al (2012) showed the benefits from removing foods with positive (allergic) reactions to IgG alone. After eliminating these foods for just 90 days, **subjects had significant reductions in weight, body mass index, waist & hip circumferences, plus reduction in blood pressure.**

Another profound study recently examined food allergen testing and elimination, in a double-blind study.

(Double-blind means neither the patients nor the prescribing doctor knew whether the patient was eating a true elimination diet or just a mock placebo diet. Clinical research means that it tests to see if there is a significant change or difference between treatment and a control where there is no treatment.)

In that 30-day study, the patients who were treated with the food allergen-elimination diet, later showed a significant change in BMI, body composition (fat % and mass) and they also showed decreased symptoms like high blood pressure. The subjects who ate a placebo diet (without the food allergens eliminated) had no change.

A recent study tested the white blood cell (leukocyte) reactions to 237 foods (Ali et al 2017). This was a double-blind, controlled trial which showed significant improvement in the global improvement scale for the IBS patients who eliminated consumption of the low-level food allergens. Scientists and clinicians have found that the same inflammatory food reactions which cause GI (gastral system) symptoms in other diseases also contribute to obesity.

**A study by Willis et al (2018) examined the benefits of eliminating food allergens by themselves in comparison to food allergen elimination plus all the protocols described in this book.** The study published in *Food Science and Nutrition Research*, showed that all subjects who had food allergen elimination (ALCAT testing methods) showed significant changes. However the combination of food allergen elimination plus Dr. Willis' PAN-5 system had 75% greater weight loss (-12.4 kg), 60% greater body fat reduction, and a greater BMI reduction (-3.6 BMI).

Figure 2. Study Results

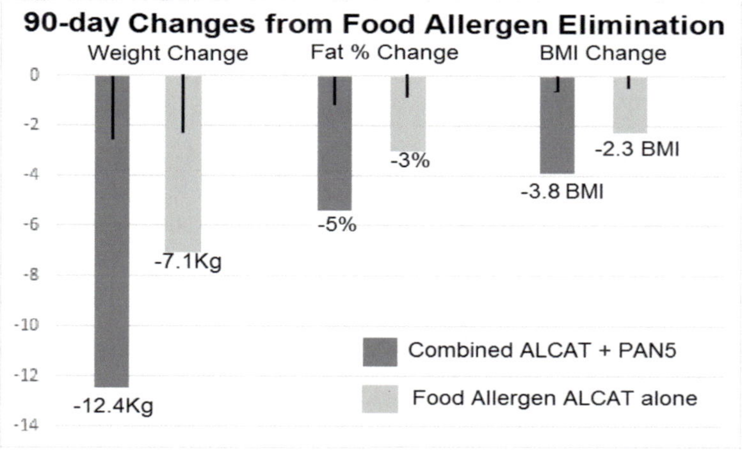


In a follow up study, the ***"Financial Savings from Obesity Reduction***" was examined. The NIH estimates that obesity (BMI > 30) yields an average $1400/year greater cost in healthcare expenses. However, these patients averaged -$1900 savings in the 12 months following obesity reduction, (Willis et al 2019).

**Menopause and Low T**

Menopause is a condition that decreases estrogen levels, which in turn, causes a decreased metabolic rate. For women who were already overweight, this also increases the risk for high blood pressure, heart disease, and type II diabetes, just to name a few diseases. Luckily, this weight loss method is effective in raising metabolism for these people too. The collection of different protocols in this treatment plan will increase your energy and vitality while also dropping blood pressure and HbA1c! (Actually 90% of my patients who came with Type II Diabetes left after one year with normal, healthy HbA1c test results.)

Right now, 60% of Americans don't exercise regularly and 73% of Americans are overweight. Please read that again. So if we all exercised would we all be skinny? Obviously exercise is not the answer to this disease but it contributes significantly to raise the metabolism and reduce the fat. **The Aerobic-surge exercise will increase muscle density, which will raise your metabolism. (**See chapter 5.) Aerobic-surges, plus small portion-size meals, will increase fat consumption, and natural foods will raise your metabolism as well.

This is the PAN-5 formula that you will read more about in future chapters.

The total daily duration of the Aerobic-surges when performing five/day is just 10 total minutes, and it has been shown more effective in fat loss than going to the gym for an hour each day! Daily Aerobic-surge exercises will also benefit you by providing:

- Decreased risk of osteoporosis
- Decreased risk of cardiovascular heart disease
- Decreased blood pressure
- Decreased depression (increases and maintains serotonin levels)
- Decreased LDL, cholesterol, and triglycerides.
- Improved insulin sensitivity (type II diabetes can been cured)
- Increased effective bowel movements
- Reduced risk of breast cancer
- Improved overall health

Many people say they “lack of time” for exercise and that is there the 2-minute Aerobic-surge will help. A recent study by Grossman et al (*Menopause* 2017) showed that women who were prescribed a brief, high intensity interval training (HIIT) program were 50% more compliant than women prescribed a longer duration of walking every day.

**Exercise helps reduce the symptoms of menopause**. Perez/Lopez et al completed a systematic review study (which is a study of numerous studies). In 11 studies examined, 1943 women (ages 45 – 65 who were not on hormone therapy), had a significant reduction in symptoms from exercise alone. The two-minute Aerobic-surge exercise will provide you with an effective method of reducing postmenopausal symptoms without requiring hours in the gym.

Have you seen advertisements for treatment of "Low T" (low testosterone)? This is a valid, measurable deficit that can be examined quickly, with a two-minute blood drawn for testosterone and thyroid hormone tests.

**Testosterone is an anabolic steroid that is needed for women too.** Not only does testosterone play a vital role in restoring current muscles cells (which is needed continually), but it is also important in laying down the matrix for strong bones. In women, decreased testosterone has been found significant in osteoporosis. So we all need an optimal balance of testosterone. We'll need your primary care physician (PCP) to test to determine if you have a deficit in testosterone. They may prescribe treatment with weekly injections or oral medication.

Our body cells are constantly being destroyed and rebuilt. A deficit in testosterone reduces the efficacy in that process and disrupts the ideal balance and density of muscle, bone, and connective tissue like ligaments. **Fat is needed for building cells,** particularly cell walls, but increased deposits in the fat cells may associated with metabolic depression in obesity. This is very common in hypothyroid secretion too.

Thyroid hormone production is initiated by thyroid stimulating hormone (TSH). When thyroid hormones T3 and T4 are low, then the TSH is high, calling for a greater production of these cells. Hypothyroid secretion can be caused by many things from genetics to diet and environment. Whatever the cause, a low balance of thyroid hormones also causes weight gain. This is one common cause of metabolic depression and could be your cause. Ask your PCP for testing of your thyroid and testosterone levels.

***Digest this*:** Hidden food allergies are often the cause of the overweight disease (90% of my patients had reactions to over 20% of the 250 foods tested). Just eliminating this cause by itself will help but combining all of the protocols I am describing will help it happen faster and in greater volumes of fat reduction!

# SECTION II

# CHAPTER 5

# Ignite Your Metabolism!

**Taste of Victory**: Amy saw the success of patients who were treated at my Rightsize clinic and it inspired her to work toward losing weight. She described that she was never able to lose the "pregnancy fat" even though she exercised and "watched what she ate". I had her complete a nutritional assessment and noticed that she was eating healthy food, but at almost six hour intervals (6am – noon – 7pm). I also observed that her exercise was too intense. So I taught her how to ride her bicycle in the Aerobic Threshold (which is the only time the body uses fat as the primary fuel), and I also told her to eat Six times a day.

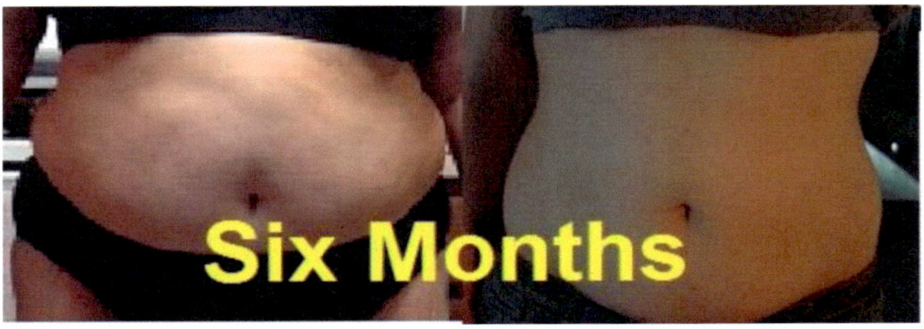


At first her children laughed, but they later thought it was fun that she could eat six times a day and they joined her routine. When she exercised, she decreased her training intensity and bought a Polar® heart rate monitor. She recorded her immediate HR and the average HR for each duration of training. After three months, Amy had lost 30 pounds and 10 inches from her waist! Her husband, Ray, was a bit envious and joined in her program. Together they lost a total of 90 pounds and have started several of their friends in the RightSize weight loss program!

## Two-Minute, Aerobic-Surge exercises

**A quick 2-minute "aerobic energy surge" (Aerobic-surge) will increase your metabolism and help you burn more fat.** It's ideal if we perform this exercise right before each of our meals or snacks every three hours. Here are 30 easy exercises that won't make you sweat, but should reach your target heart rate (HR) in the Aerobic Threshold (75% of max HR).

The mathematical estimate of your aerobic threshold is (220- age) x .75. First, please consult your primary care physician and allow them to share in celebrating your success later. If you become lightheaded or dizzy after such an exercise bout then you need to stop, because you may have other health care needs that must be addressed.

These easy exercises and try them all over the next few weeks to see which challenge you and become your favorite exercises to accelerate your metabolism. If your heart rate is not elevated to that level, you can certainly use the exercise in regular training, but it will *not* count as your intndense Aerobic-surge exercise.

## Ab Crunches

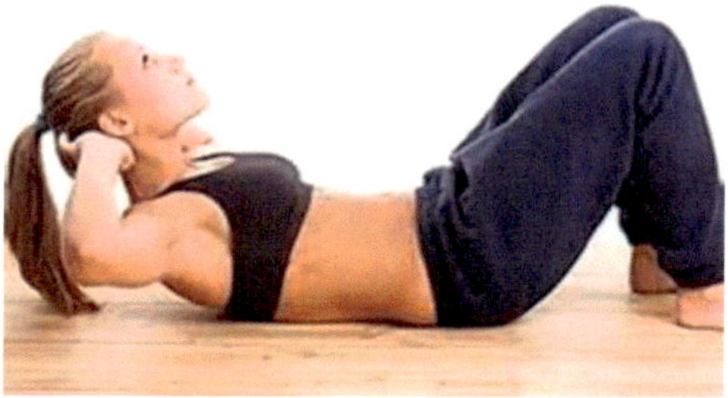

These are the classic abdominal maneuver where you lay on your back and bring your knees slightly toward your shoulders. (Don't crane your neck!) "Pull your body together" and hold for two seconds. The total duration should be 120 seconds and you should feel you HR elevated after the first 45 seconds.

## Arm Pedal

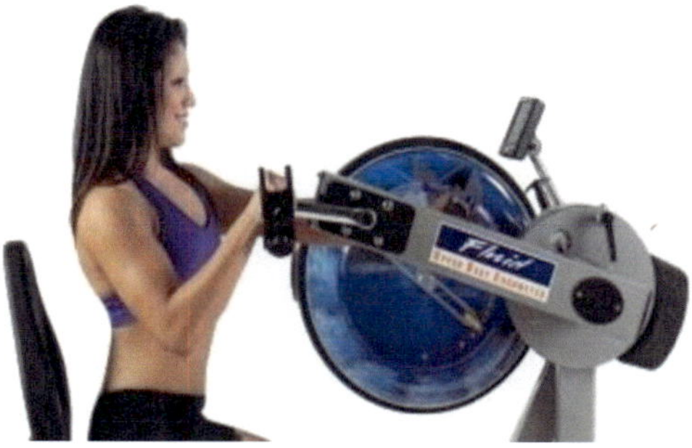

You can use one of the inexpensive arm ergometer cycles and use your hands/arms for the power to rotate the cycle instead of your feet/legs. I always suggest the bicycle over treadmill so the weight is in the "saddle" (seat) but this is even better and we rarely use our arms continually so this is an easy tool to raise the heart rate. (We also used this device to help the Shriners pediatric burn patients gain strength and they loved it because their legs may have been too badly injured to use a treadmill or bicycle.)

## Ball Pushups

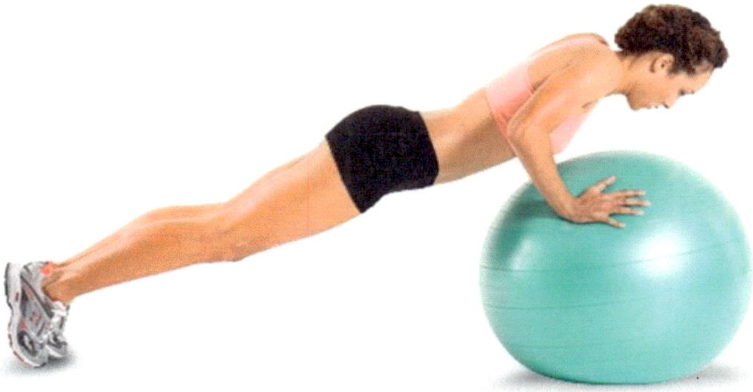

My Favorite! Strat slow and if you can accomplish 30 ball pushups, then switch to 30 crunches, followed by 30 pushups and 30 crunches. Then tell me when you can do 120 straight ball pushups and you'll hear my *"Hooyah!"* all the way from Galveston.

## Back Row

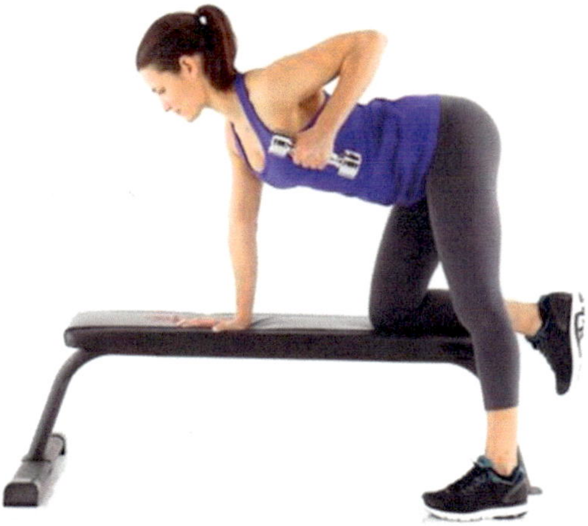

For a simple back exercise:

- Kneel one leg onto a chair along with the stability of one hand (same side as the knee). – Grab a dumbbell (DB) with the other hand and lower it almost all of the way to the ground.
- Lift the weight up as far as you can toward your ribs. Exhale as you lift the weight each of the 20 reps per side and then rotate light, right left right. This exercise will activate many of the different back, shoulder, and triceps muscles.

## Bicycle Sprint

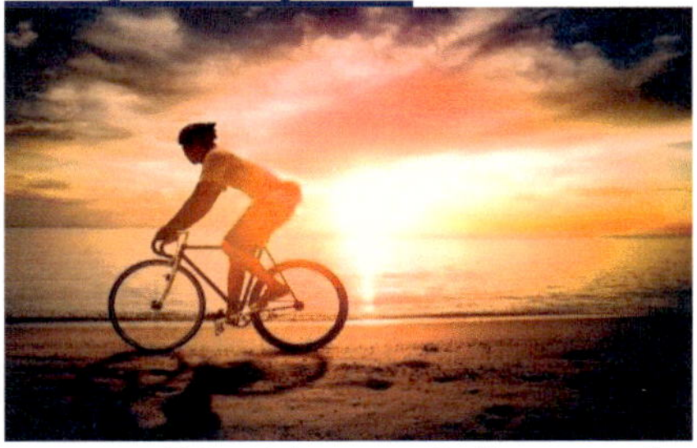

Start by pedaling as fast as you can for 60 revolutions and then just coast back! If you want to stay in the Aerobic surge for 20 minutes it equals two.

# Bed Drape/Heel Raises

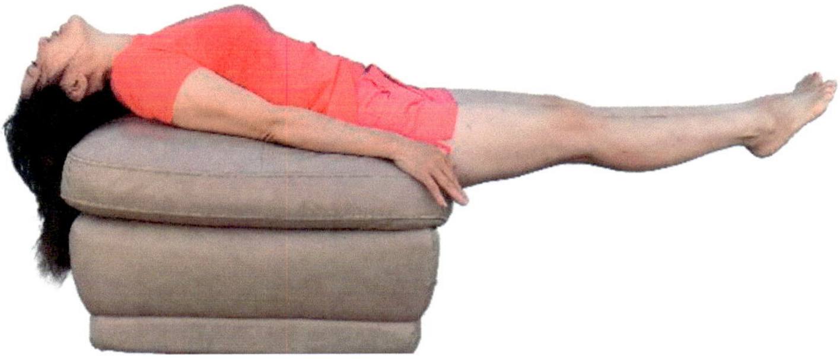

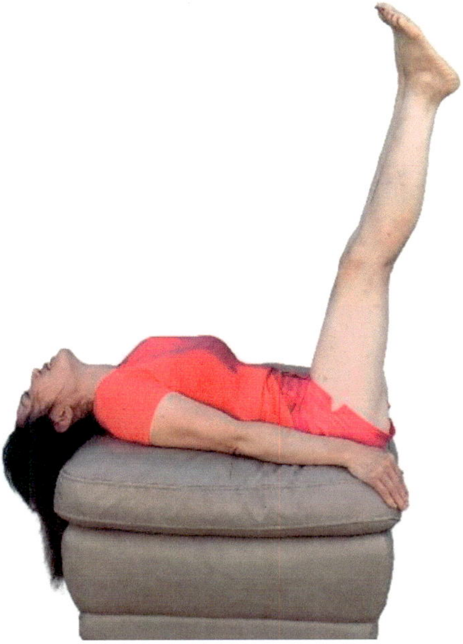

This is a unique, excellent home exercise that targets your abdominal muscles. Lay back with head to hips on the bed and let a bit of your glute muscles (butt) hang slightly over with your legs. Now straighten your legs (like a plank) and then raise your heels slowly to the sky with your knees locked in extension. Lower your legs until parallel with the floor and lift your legs again.

## Biceps Curls

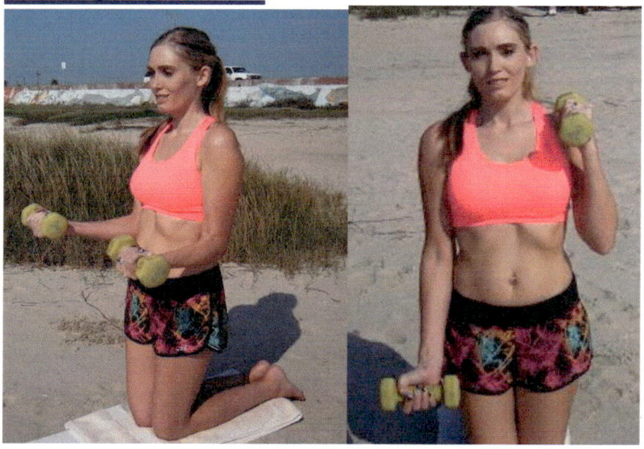

Stand and hold dumbbells in the supine position (as if you are holding a soup bowl) and fully curl your fist towards your chin while you keep your elbows locked against your side. Do this flat curl 20 repetitions per side rotating until you can't do any more or after 120 seconds.

## Brain Busters

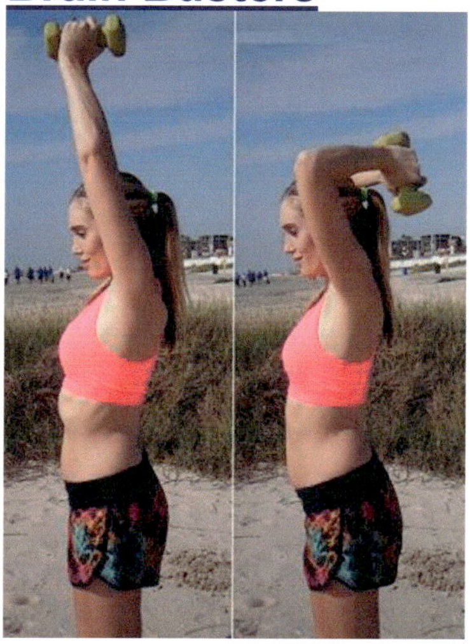

Brain-busters is a triceps exercise that can be performed with two dumbbells or two full 16-ounce cans or bottles of water. Stand and simply touch your fingers to the back of your head and then extend the bottle or DB until your arms are straight. Start with 100.

## Burpees!

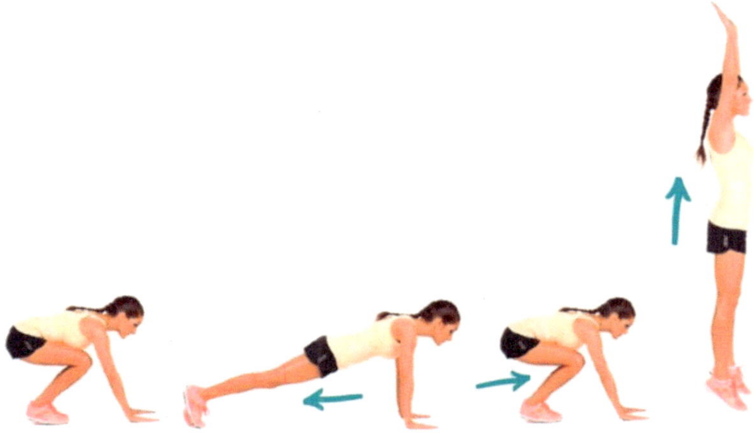

Start standing with your feet 18” apart. Now bend down to touch your hands to the ground before extending your feet back for the “push up” position, Then reverse and jump up.

## Calf Raises

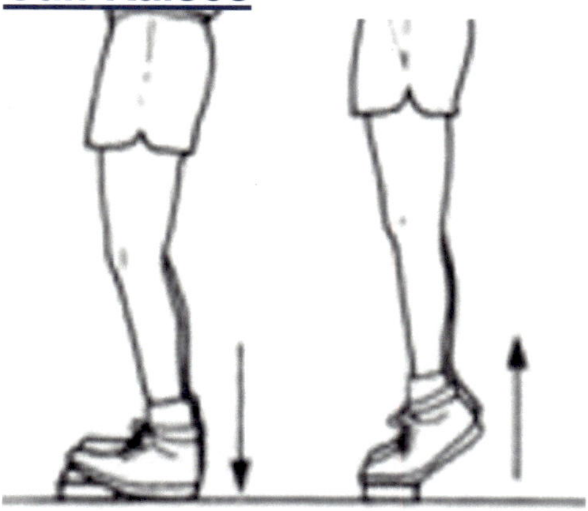

The calf muscle (gastrocnemius) has medial and lateral heads. To activate this muscle safely, get a 2x4 board and place it on the ground, or stand on a stair step with a hand rail. Now hold ontop the rail with one hand and hold a DB in the other hand. Raise your heel and tighten your abs. Trade foot and hand holding weight for another 60 reps.

## Clock Swings

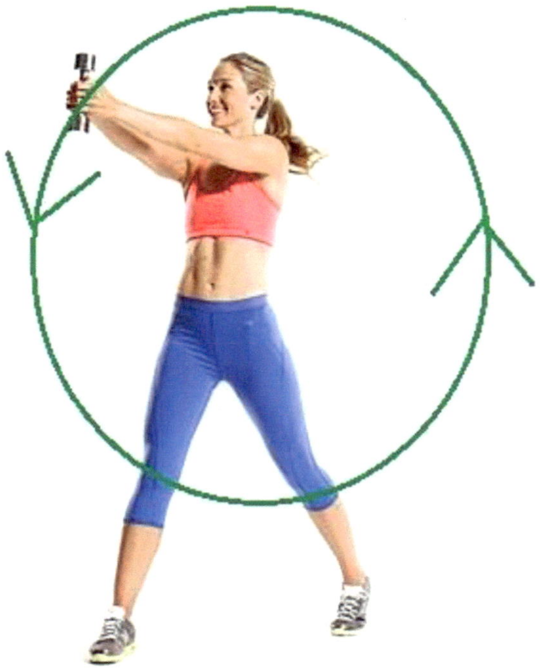

Grab a dumbbell and slowly rotate it through the clock rotation 1 o'clock to 12 o'clock. Then reverse the clock and target 5-second stops at 12 to 6 and then 9 to 3 o'clock. . Keep the muscle tone high and you'll likely feel your back and abdominal muscles working too. That's a good thing!

## Curl a Child!

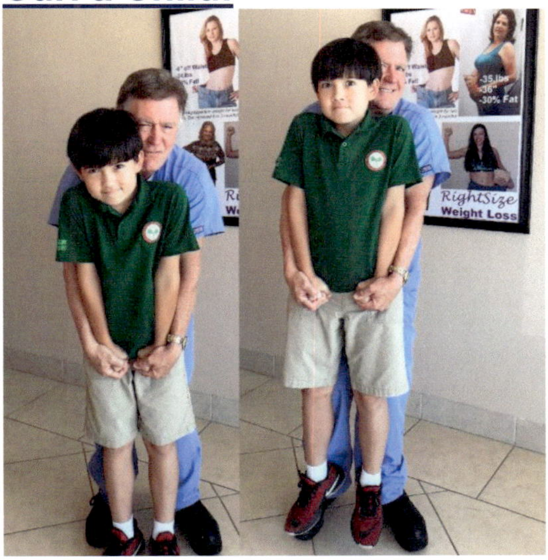


Yes Aaron thinks this is funny but it will get your HR up!

## Downward-Facing Dog

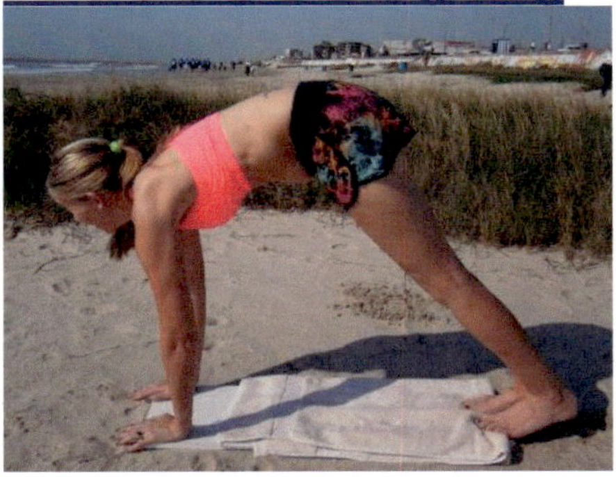

Start with your hands and knees touching the ground in a "push up" position. Then walk your feet and hands up until your hips are to heaven. Now go from the flat, tummy-down position to the flexed "dog" position 50 times.

## Duck Walk:

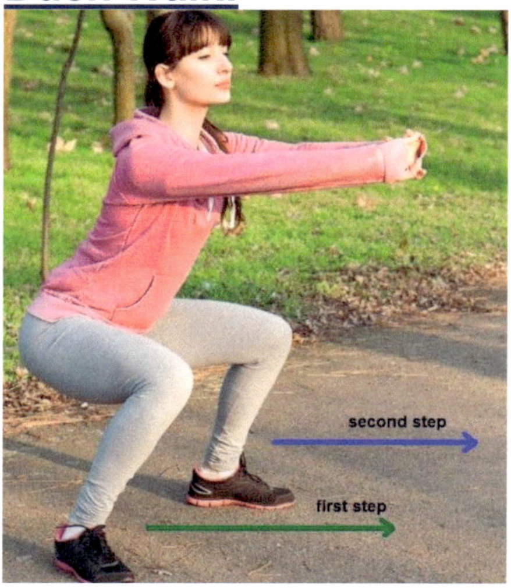


Squat, and walk one foot at a time as you STAY Squatted!

## Forward Lunge:

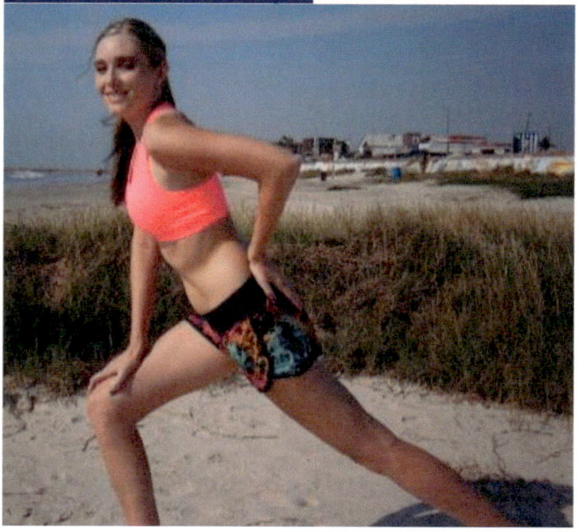

With your body in the upright position, simply take a long step out and bend the front knee to a 45 degree angle while the other leg is extended. For the energy surge, complete a brisk 30 lunges out (60 seconds) and 30 lunges returning to your original position.

## Frog Jump

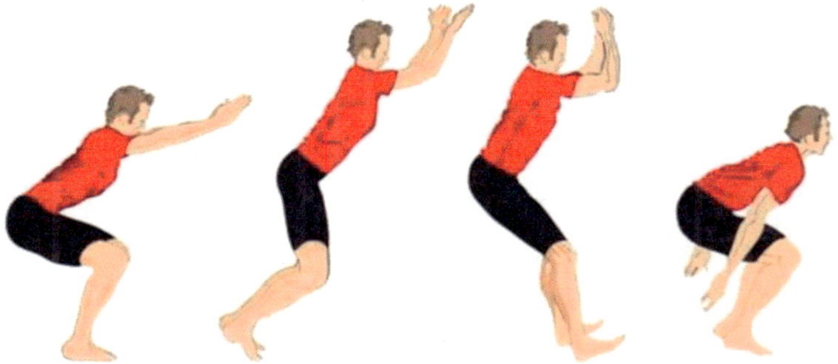

This is actually a plyometric exercise where one muscle group goes from full extension (longest) to full contraction (shortest). Squat as low as you can and then swing your arms to Jump Forward! (Squat pops are just straight up.)

## Hip Lifts

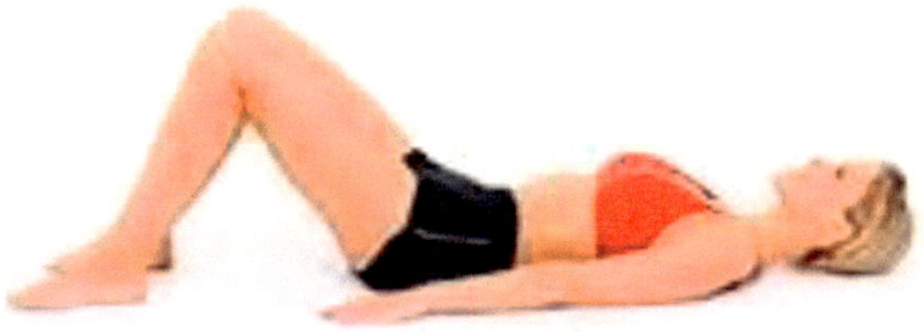

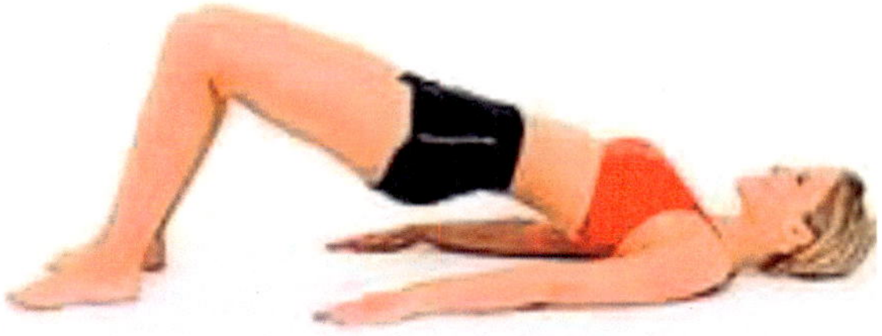

You will do the next set of exercises on your exercise pad or bed (remove all sheets and blankets). Lay supine (tummy up) on the floor and place a laptop computer or a baby on your tummy. Then feel the back of your legs as you push your heels down and raise your hips 6-12 inches. (This exercise is actually better on the floor if you are comfortable there.)

Exhale as you lift your hips 120 times.

## Incline Chest Press

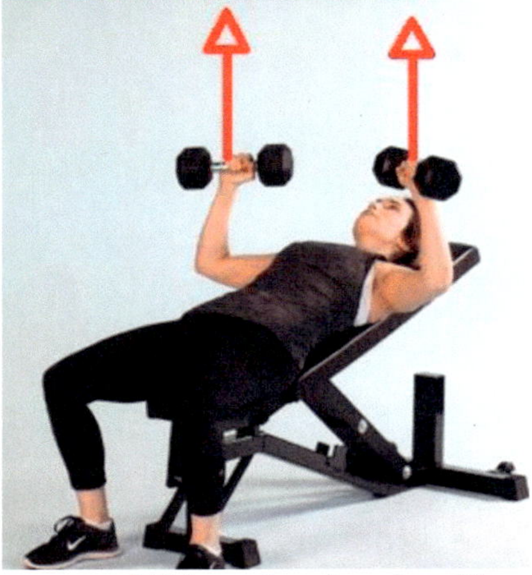

Sit leaning back with a two-pound DB in each hand; bring your hands from your chest to as high as possible. Use hammer grip (palms facing in) and the rotate to thumbs facing in for 120 total.

## Jumping Jacks

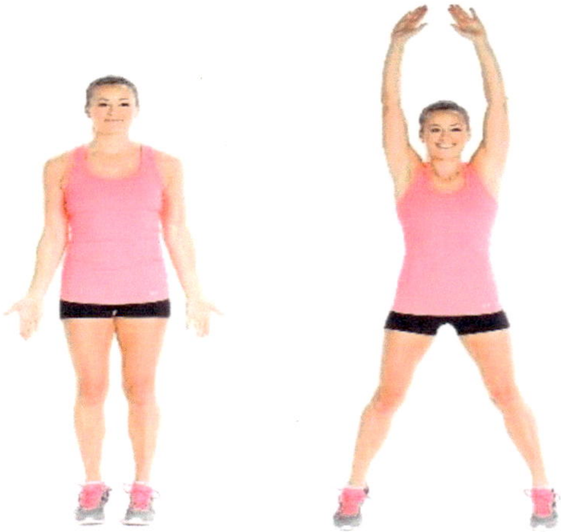


Start with both legs together and your hands by your sides. Hop both legs away from each other (24"), clapping your hands above your head, then jump to bring your heels together, slapping the sides of your thighs. Two minutes is your goal at 75% of your max HR.

## Mountain Climber

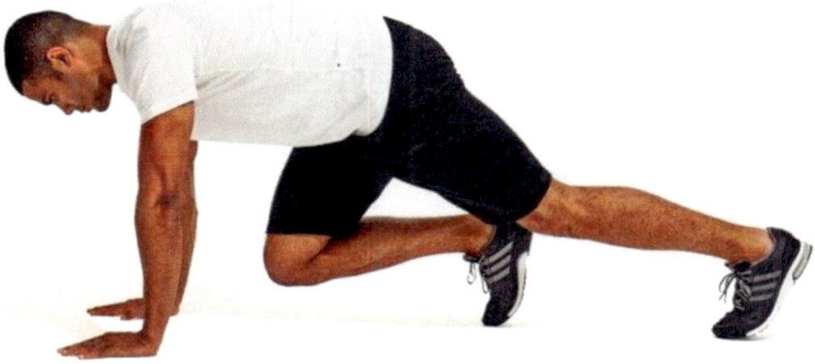

Simply take a "Push up" stance and alternate bringing each knee to your chest. Head Up & Butt Down!

## Milk Shakes

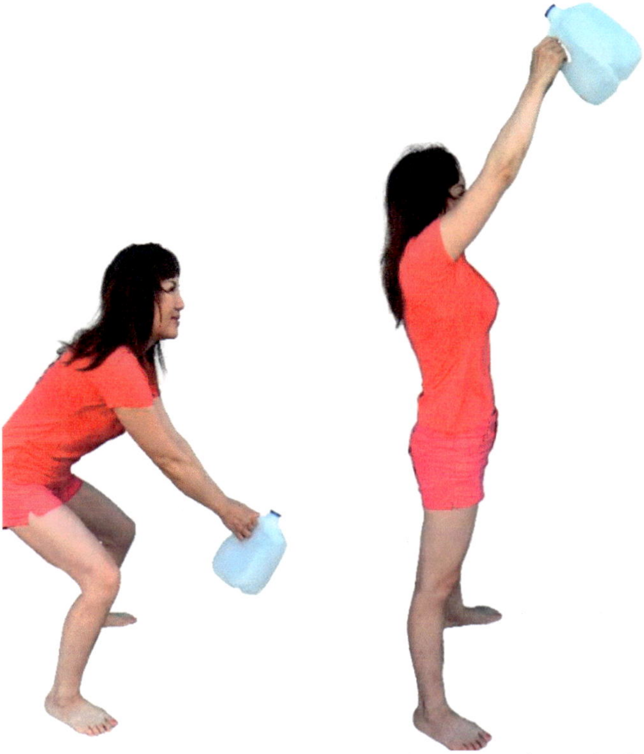

Grab a gallon of milk (or water) and shake from ground to overhead as fast as you can for two minutes (Floor to Ceiling)!

## Push-Ups

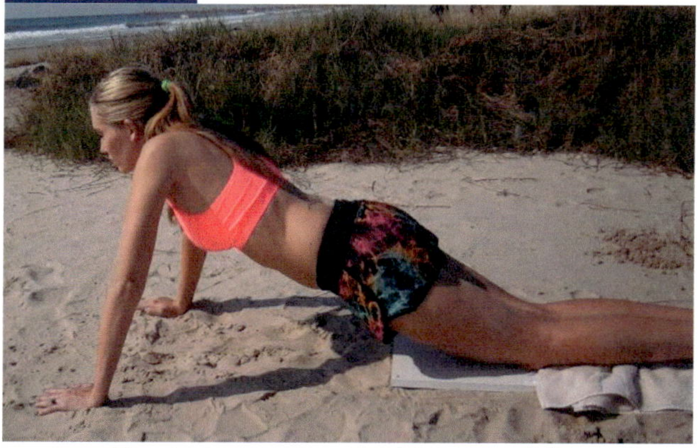

Push-ups are an old school favorite, but holding your body in a solid plank while you lower your chest to the ground activates many muscles as stabilizers as well. Women start with your knees on the ground. Two minutes of pushups will be a great success.

## Reverse Plank Walk-Around

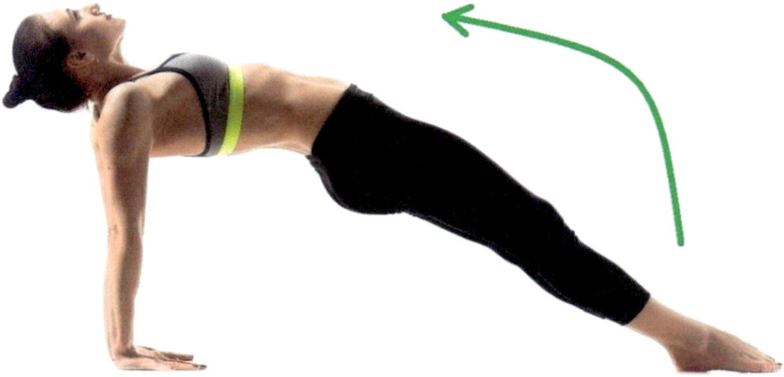

Start laying on your back and press up with your arms. First just hold your body in this reverse plank position and then in a few days shuffle your feet around to the left to make a full circle.

## Roll Ups

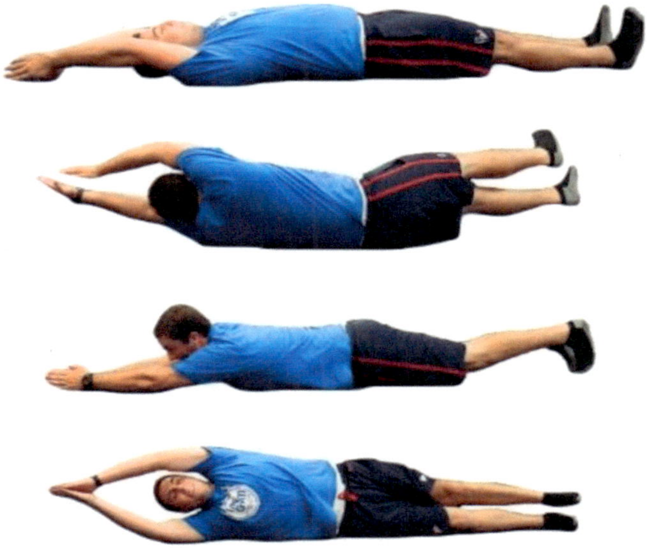

Lay on your back (supine) with your arms and legs extended. Roll your body and then roll back! This sounds simple enough, but you'll be surprised when you take your heart rate after doing this 100 times!

## Scissors Kicks

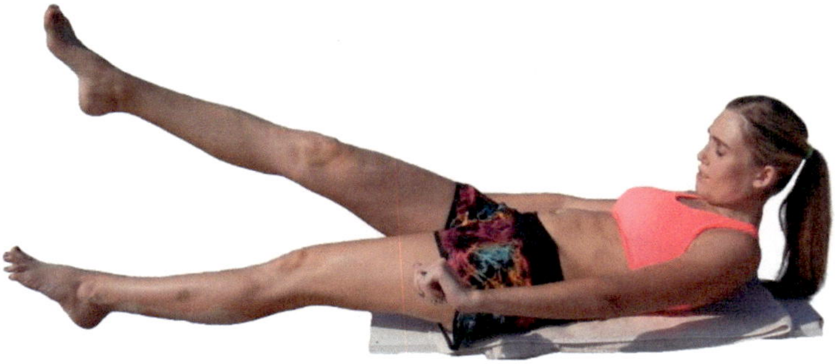

Lay on your back and simply keep your legs elevated while you are alternately raising left leg while lowering the right leg. Keep your legs stiff.

## Shoulders Extension

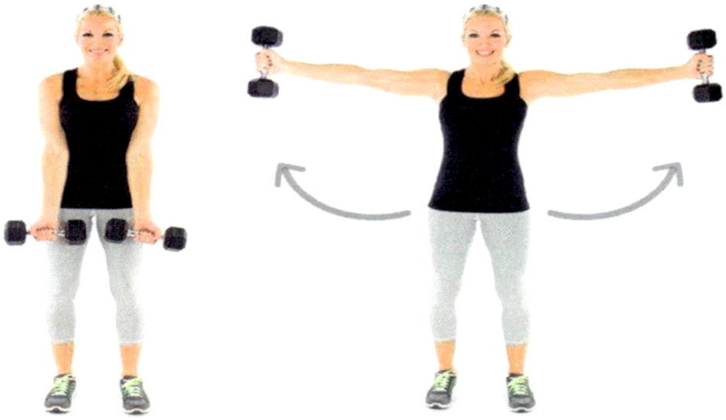

Grab a can of food or a light dumbbell and perform 100 repetitions. If you get tired after 50 reps, set your cans down and perform 50 scissor kicks to keep your heart rate elevated before you finish the can lifts! Lift the dumbbells with Hammer grip or supine, flat grip. (Exhale on the way up.)

## Side Scissor

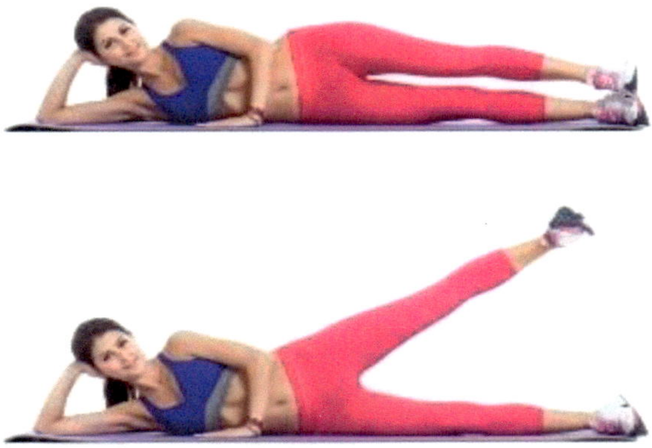

Lay on your side and raise your top leg as high as you can while keeping your leg stiff, 60 lifts for each leg = victory!

## Side Plank Hip Elevation

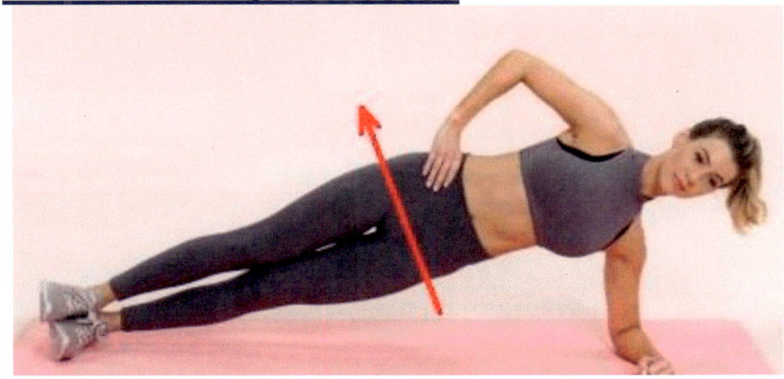

This is similar to the "Side Torso Lift," but on your right side with your right elbow bent to be directly under your shoulder. Now instead of focusing on your torso, raise your hips "to heaven." Keep your knees bent slightly and your legs touching. Tighten your abdominal muscles each time you raise your hips and keep your head in alignment with your spine.

## Skipping

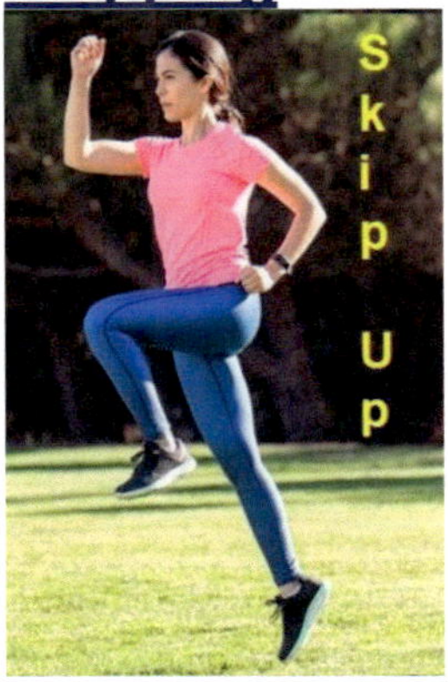


As you jog surge one knee high and after landing then surge the next knee high.

## Squats

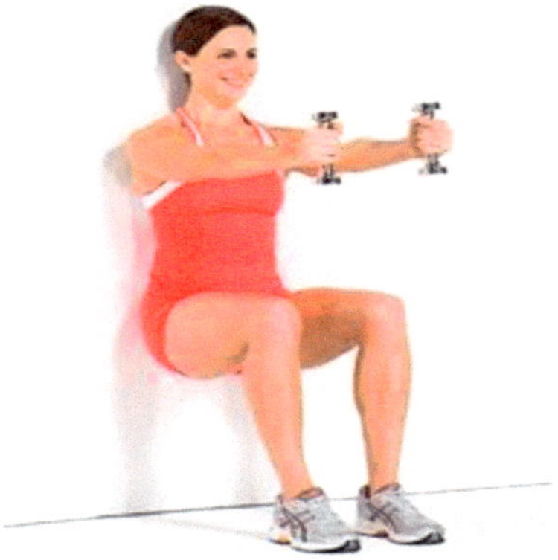

Hold a 2-pound dumbbell (DB) in each hand and with your back to a smooth wall, simply squat down 50 times. In doing this maneuver, make sure to inhale on the way down and exhale on the way back up (Blow yourself up). You should try to squat to a depth where your knees are bent to 45 degrees. Keep your head straight.

## Squat Pops

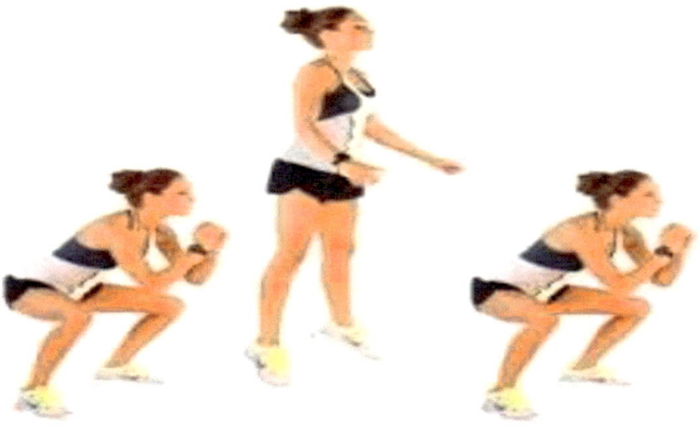

At first you can hold onto a rail and slowly squat as low as you can, then quickly pop back up with enough force that your feet slightly leave the ground.

## Stair Climber.

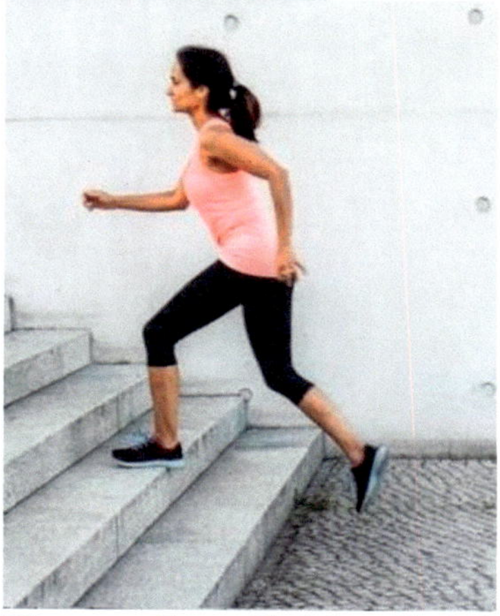

Run up four flights of stairs (there times = 120 steps) at the office.

## Squiggle Jumps

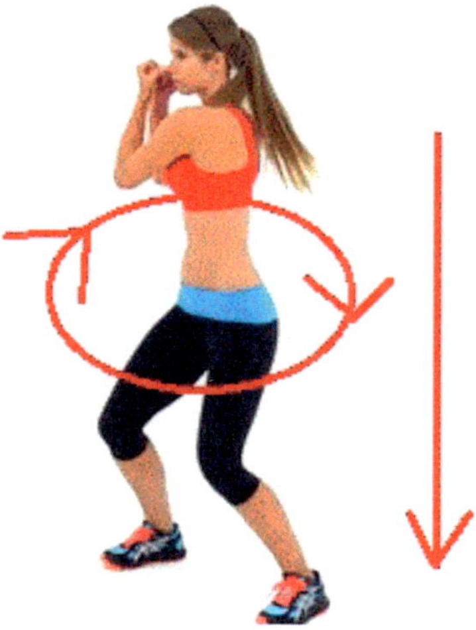

These are a unique and popular aerobic-surge today. Kids love this because they can honestly beat adults when competing. Start by simultaneously doing two to three hip twists as you squat down with your butt in your heels, and then jump up! Do this for two minutes. This is an excellent energy surge to perform on work breaks.

## Super-Woman

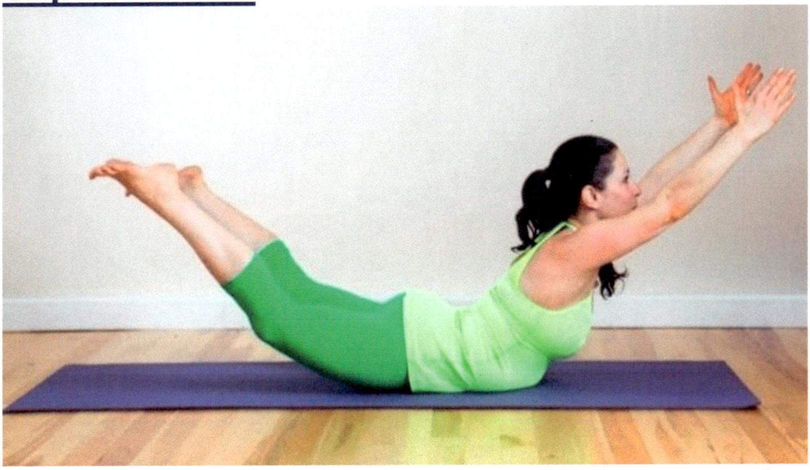

These are the endurance exercise that you perform by laying down prone (face to the ground) and simultaneously lifting up your arms and heels. Hold this pose for two minutes <u>after</u> your heart and breathing rate are elevated.

## Toes to the Sky

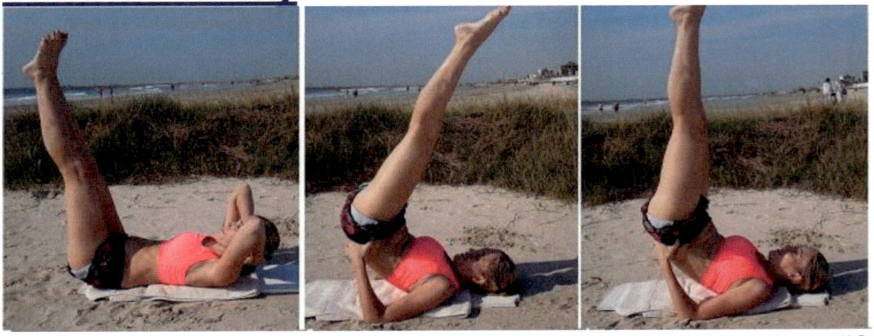

Lie on your back with your legs straight up, then lift your hips and reach your toes to the sky. You will have to work consciously to elevate your heart with this exercise. Keep your ab muscles tight the whole 2 minutes while you do 100 repetitions.

## Trot

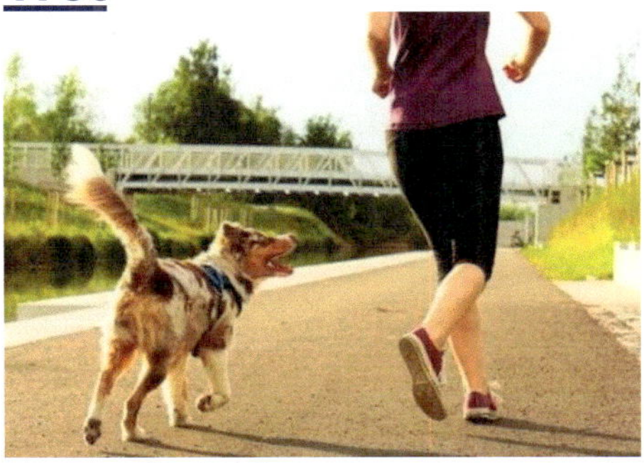

Briskly around your house with alternating steps and jumps. Trot like a thoroughbred with step – step – hop, step – step – hop, which keeps alternating the leg used to propel you upwards. Do it with yuour kids for silly fun.

## V-Tucks

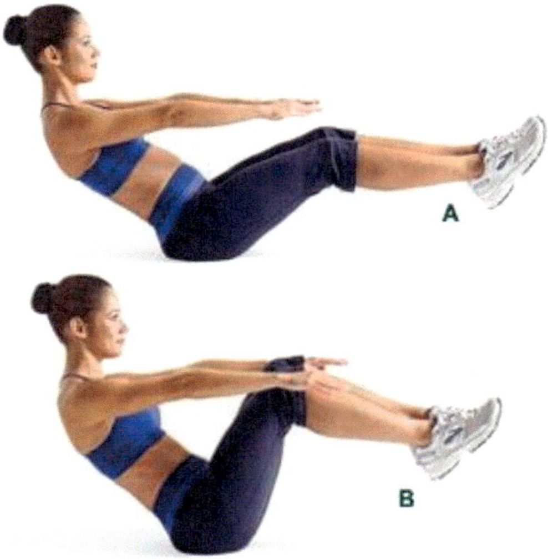


Sit on your butt with your knees and feet extended (just above the floor). Bring your knees to your chest, exhaling on the way. You can also “super set” this with other exercises without stopping.

## Walk on All Fours (Bear Crawls)

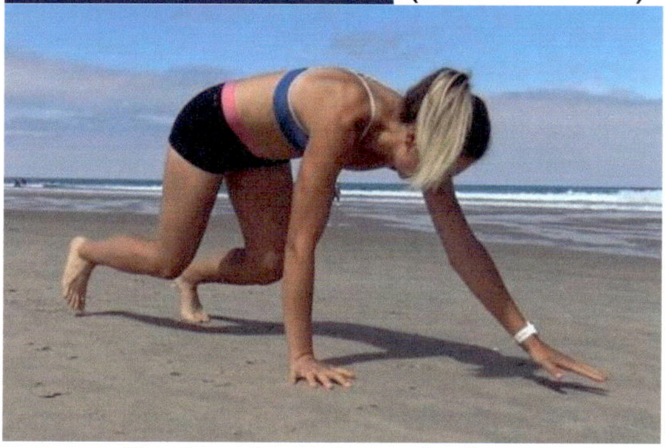

Pretend you're a baby again and walk on all fours with your hips and head Up! (Athletes call this a Bear Crawl but babies call it "moving all up!")

## Water Walks

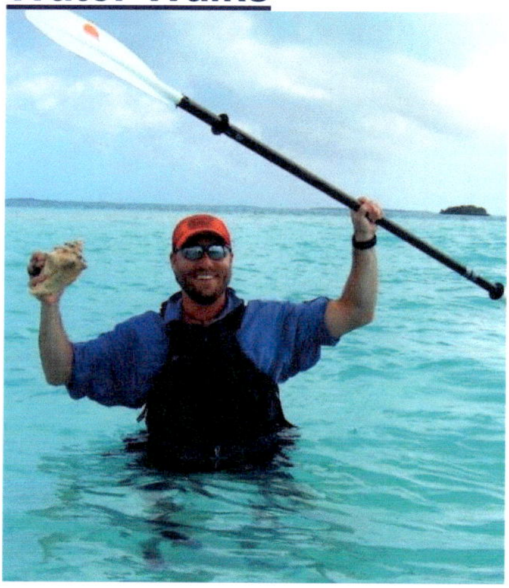

In the ocean or a pool, walk briskly through the water with stiff legs that make resistance when you are swinging your legs.

***Digest this*: *START SLOWLY!*** If you have not exercised in a few months, it is not reasonable that you can start off performing the challenging exercises 5/day.

# Chapter 6
# Tease, Don't Deny Yourself!

**Taste of Victory**: "Buzz" is an avid golfer and enjoys traveling. He came to me with only symptoms of slowed metabolism. When we tested for food allergies, he actually had acute to light reactions to 105 of the 250 foods tested. Like many people, his success has varied from one month to the next. However his long term success has included a 23% change in his total body fat in just 3 months! This is a long-term journey that he is obviously enjoying. You too can lose weight on a cruise!

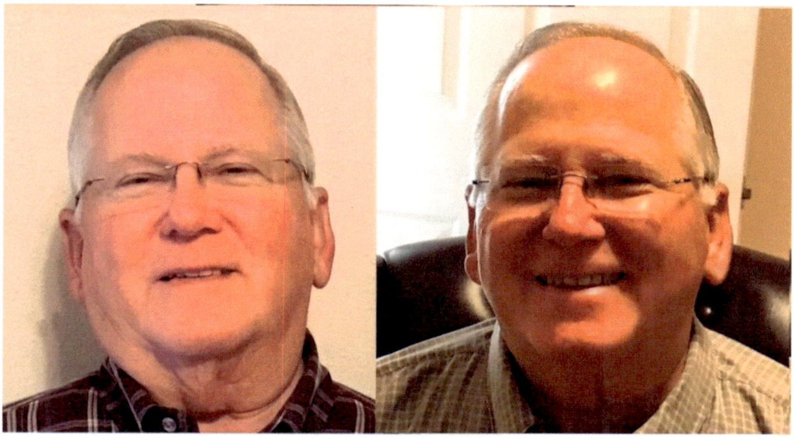

**30-Day Change (-16lbs and -14% Fat )**

**Teasing your body will help you to gain a faster metabolic rate! Here are simple, proven tips to raise your metabolism:**

**Move First** thing in the morning. It has been shown in abundant studies that performing a quick exercise routine when you first wake up accelerates the metabolism for a few hours. While it is still elevated, do other things to keep the metabolic rate as high as possible, like eating natural foods.

**One Bite ASAP**. Eating one bite of fruit or meat upon waking will significantly elevate the metabolism. When we sleep, the body is fasting and has the lowest metabolic level. Eating just one bite is a tease that turns up the fire on your metabolism. Eat one bite immediately after your first exercise and then leisurely get ready for work before having a full breakfast. (Skipping breakfast keeps the metabolism running at a slower pace.)

**Eat Breakfast** because fasting throws your body into survival mode, where metabolic rate and energy are significantly reduced. "Tell your body" that it will have ample food throughout the day so that it keeps the fires burning as high as possible!

**Turn up the Heat** on your food. Capsaicin is the natural compound that makes chili peppers "hot." Eating a tablespoon of chopped red or green chili peppers achieves a temporary spike in the metabolism up to 23%. Drs. Shin and Moritani (2007) found in their study that consuming capsaicin, green tea, and chicken essence tablets raised the "thermogenic effect" by triggering a metabolic "fight or flight" response, which raised the basal metabolic rate without increasing heart rate or blood pressure. Eat some chili peppers on your burger or add red peppers on pizza for a bit of metabolic heat.

**Ladies Pump Iron** because iron deficiency causes the metabolism to plummet. If you have low iron, your body will carry less oxygen to the muscles; then the less efficient muscle activity will lower the basal metabolic rate as a protection mechanism. So eat more beans, dark leafy greens like spinach, bok choy, and broccoli.

**Go Fish** or at least consume more fish or fish oil vitamins to increase your metabolism. Several studies have shown that consuming six grams of fish oil vitamins can increase weight loss and accelerate weight loss with exercise.

**Eat High Energy Foods** like whole grains, beans, vegetables, and fruits. The higher quality "fuel" you consume, the stronger and higher the metabolic "flame."

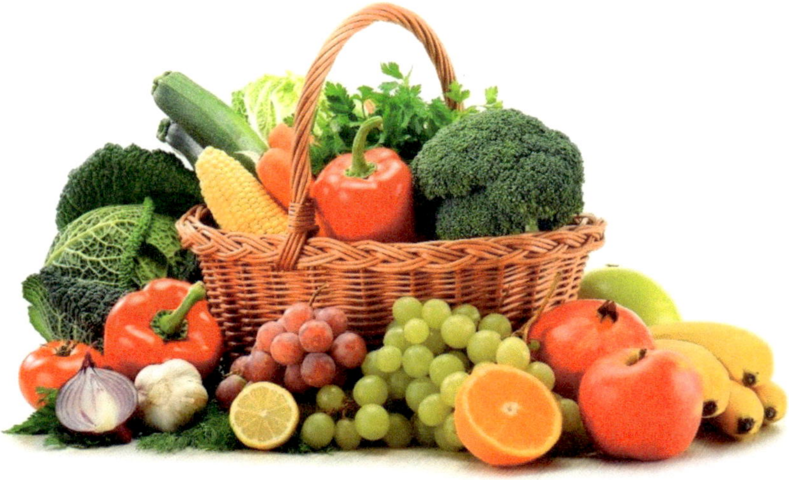

**Water for Weight Loss** was evaluated in a clinical study. It showed that subjects who drank eight glasses per day versus four glasses per day, lost more weight. Too much water can "wash out your success!" Drinking too much water causes hyponatremia (low sodium in the blood), which contributes to congestive heart failure, kidney and liver failures, and pneumonia.

**Snack Attacks** are GOOD if they are signals from your body to eat more good fuel. Throw out the chips and Snickers and pick up an apple or banana every two to three hours. This will keep you from being hungry and will keep the metabolic "fire" high.

**Protein for Lunch** is good. A pyramid sequence of eating the most nutrient dense proteins (and the largest volume < 2 cups) in the middle of your day has been used for many years. If you were not focused on portion size or exercise, then you could eat sequentially increasing and decreasing food volumes like 8 oz., 12 oz., 16 oz., 8 oz.

**Sip Coffee and Drink Water.** Drinking an eight-ounce glass of water after every cup of coffee has a thermogenic effect. Coffee can act as a diuretic, but following it with a cool glass of water will help negate the detrimental effects of coffee by itself.

**Fresh Brewed Green Tea** can be consumed for increased metabolism. While most studies link the increased metabolism of tea to caffeine, Dr. Duloo (2000) led a study that found that "green tea extract stimulates brown adipose tissue thermogenesis." (It burns more fat.) In an energy expenditure study comparing green tea versus caffeine versus a placebo, they concluded that green tea has thermogenic properties more powerful in fat breakdown than just the caffeine in the tea.

**Taurine** (energy drinks) can speed up your metabolism and may help burn fat. Studies have also shown that taurine helps reduce inflammatory reactions and works effectively as an antioxidant. The studies exploring increased fat breakdown with taurine are promising, like green tea and caffeine.

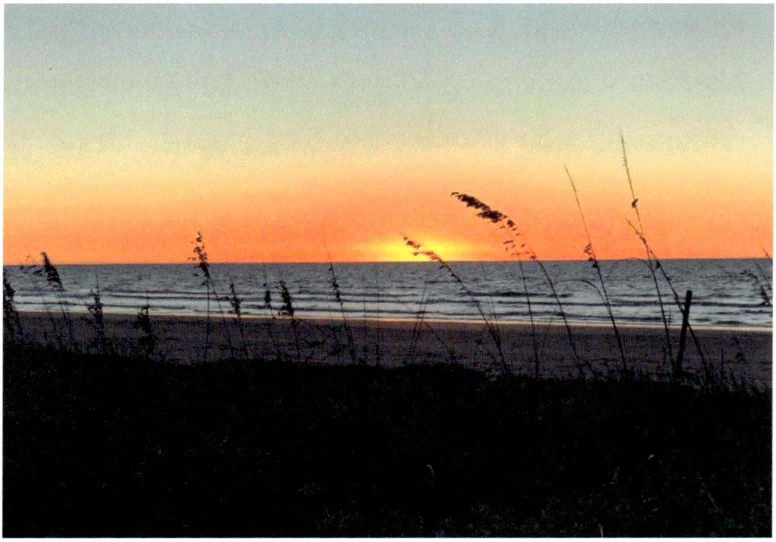

**Reducing Stress** can increase your metabolism significantly. (How can you reduce stress without the beach?) Exercise and weight loss have been shown beneficial in reducing stress, so you are on the right pathway.

Other things that can help one reduce stress are the following:

- Take Time to Breath. Schedule a few times each day to get away from noise and deeply and slowly breathe in as much air as possible, then gently exhale the air in a tiny wind-stream.
- Be Present. Shake off the past and don't worry about the future. You are here, alive, and remarkable *today*!

- Volunteer. Giving of your time to others, whether it is at church or a Big Brother/Big Sister program, it will refill you and give you joy that supersedes stress.
- Pray or Meditate. This has a centered, grounding effect and often lets one be quiet so that they can "hear" the answers to prayers. Use this time to say your mantra. "I am whole, great, and beautiful … I am whole, great, and empowered …"
- Relax. You can do numerous things to help your body relax, such as wrapping a warm towel around your neck or getting a massage. Have your special someone rub your hands and feet with a warming balm.
- Get Moving. Your energy surges don't have to be limited to just before a few meals. If your business day is stressful, take a 2-minute break to climb some stairs or walk to lunch. Exercise has been proven effective in reducing stress.
- Laugh It Up. My friend and mentor, Dr. Patch Adams, uses laughter as the best medicine! Laughter releases endorphins, which reduce stress hormones. Learn a joke or wear a squeaky red nose for no reason! That will bring

lots of quiet giggles and laughs if you just walk through a grocery store with a big red nose on! I even wore my red nose through TSA; they need laughs too!

**Sleep More.** The appetite center is in the hypothalamus of the brain, and sleep directly influences the efficacy of this organ. Leptin is the appetite suppressant hormone in the hypothalamus and Copinschi and colleagues (2014) showed that sleep deprivation decreases leptin levels, thereby raising one's appetite.

**Change Up.** Perform different aerobic surges throughout the day and try a different exercise or activity on different days. Start your morning with scissor kicks (abs) then in two to three hours, do DB curls/extensions (arms), then dash up 120 steps (legs), before you return to abs (reverse crunches), clock swings (arms/shoulders), and legs (bicycle sprint for two minutes)!

**Create Victory**. Make this "your victory" by doing what is fun and what you enjoy! Make it social to enjoy it with your family, friends, and neighbors. Invite them for a quick walk. Start the walk with the fastest speed walking cadence that raises your heart rate for two minutes, then just stroll the rest of the time.

**Feed Your Soul.** Scientific research has shown that prayer helps the patients who are praying, and prayers from others helps the people being prayed over. Why not ask for God to be your partner in this victory? Mark 11:24 says, "*Therefore I tell you, whatever you ask for in prayer, believe that you have received it, and it will be yours.*"

**Be Optimistic.** As the sun rises, tease your body into gaining a faster metabolic rate by jumping up 100 times and eating one bite of dark chocolate a few minutes before eating your first meal. Unique foods and teases help to accelerate your program. And don't forget to rotate your foods so you never eat the same foods twice in a day or two days in a row. "See" your ideal size and it will be yours again!

## ABC Healthy Foods

**Can you eat your ABC's of healthy food each week?**

**Apricots** are great, tasty treats (my petite grandmother's favorite) that increase vitamins A and C. Plus they are high in fiber, iron, and calcium.

**Apples** increase peristalsis (movement of food through the stomach and intestines); they help in detoxification and yield better digestion of complex foods.

**Asparagus is a veggie who is full of Benefits!** Not only is it packed with essential vitamins, minerals, proteins, fiber, and antioxidants, Asparagus has 57% of your Vitamin K, 18% of Vitamin A, and 12% of your Vitamin C (RDA).

It lowers blood pressure and the water rich fiber helps in weight loss (see recipes). **Plus it helps in pregnancy** by giving folate (B9) which is needed in development of the neural tube! (Plus you won't have to pee as much!)

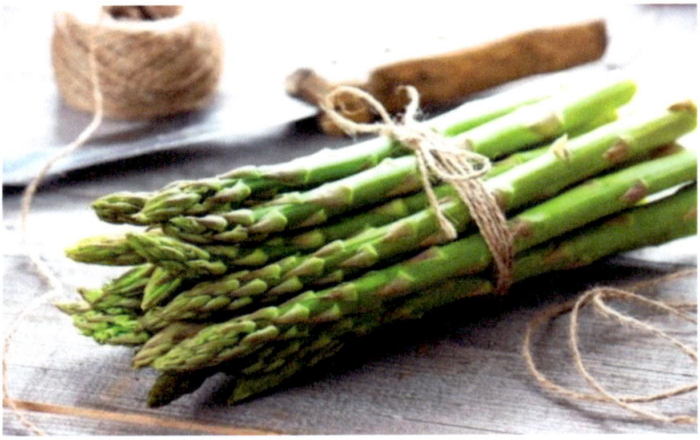

**Bananas** are not only a good treat (even though not dense with nutrients), but you can use them as a sweetener and to thicken shakes and soups!

**Beets** ≈ bind baby bind! They bind to fats, decrease water retention, and reduce colon cancer.

**Brussel sprouts** are a great source of omega-3 fatty acids, plus vitamins A, C, E, K, calcium, and iron. Try them dry roasted at 400°with a little extra virgin olive oil.

**Cabbage** - did you think this was just a useless food? It's actually loaded with vitamins K, C, B6, calcium, choline, phosphorus, selenium, niacin (B3), folate, and copper!

**Carrots** are optimal beta-carotenes that bind to cholesterol. The green diet of good foods that are not causing inflammatory reactions will also reduce blood pressure, cancer, and many other diseases besides curing obesity!

**Chili peppers** will increase metabolism. *Burn baby burn!*

**Cucumbers** are a natural diuretic and increase metabolism.

**Dates** are delicious, but watch out for added sugar. This is a good sticky ingredient used in the LARA bars that are a great, all natural snack!

**Eggplant.** Try this crustless spinach quiche and send me the picture to share with others.

**Fennel** and fennel seeds are great Mediterranean spices to add to organic recipes.

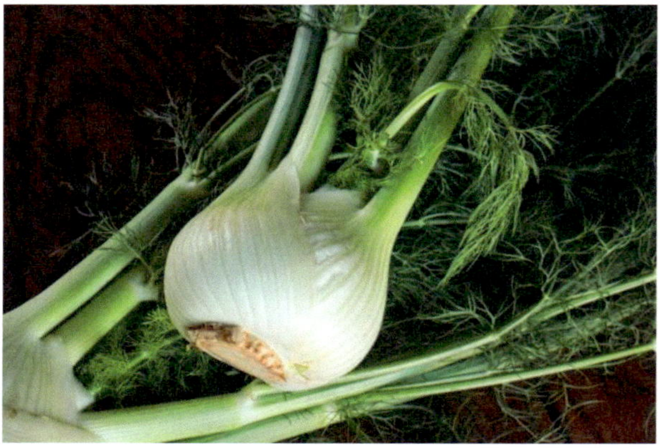

**Garlic** is also a diuretic and increases metabolism with reduction of bad bacterial growth. (It also helps keep the mosquitos away when you're working in the garden.)

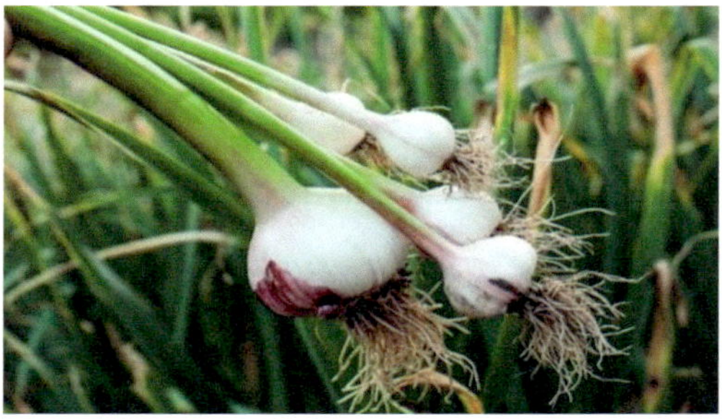

**Grapefruit** increases the metabolism and is proven to help increase fat loss.

**Green tea** increases oxidation for increased fat breakdown. (Lipton's is black tea leaf.)

**Habanero peppers** are great to raise the fire in your metabolism and good if you're allergic to jalapeños.

**Inca berries** taste like sour treats and are great to garnish foods from fruit salad to our Energy Bars!

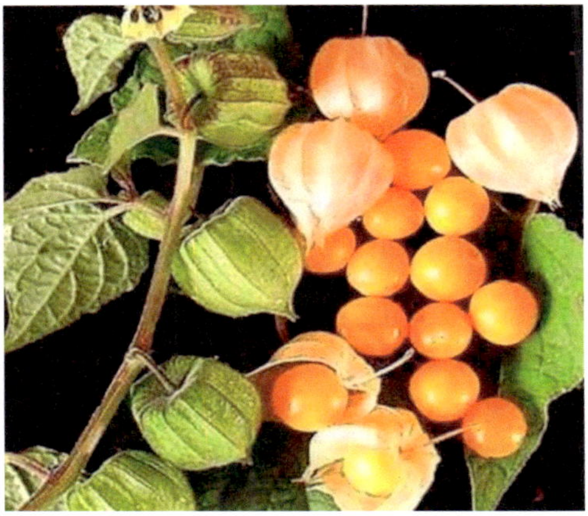

**Jalapeños** are a Texas favorite. To avoid the super-hot spice, buy the large ripe peppers, cut out the seeds, and toss in boiling water for a few seconds before eating.

**Kelp** is a great nutrient-dense, leafy vegetable. Use this as a variation from spinach or green leaf lettuce.

**Lamb** or lamb chop is a lean, delicious, nutrient-dense food. It is far better than beef for cholesterol and while it is higher in calories, that means better, long-term fuel in a delicious food!

**Lychee** is a fruit that has been shown beneficial in weight loss, plus lowers blood pressure. It grows wild in China and was originally used to flavor cocktails. Dried lychee can be added to morning shakes of fresh fruits for a different texture and aroma

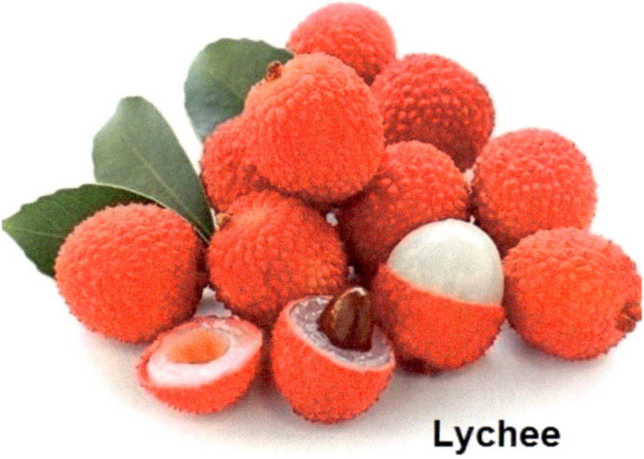

**Lychee**

**Miso** is made from fermented soybeans and boasts different flavors that are tasty while increasing the fat burn: Shiro (white) is sweet, ala (red) is salty, and lanka is yellow and salty.

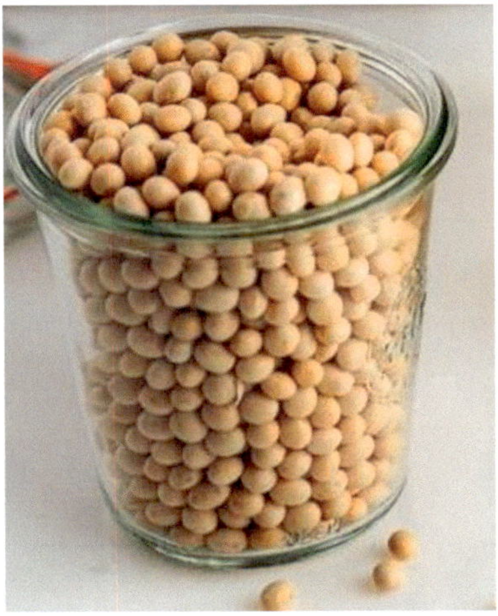

**Nectarines** are great antioxidants with carotenoids, vitamin C, iron, and phosphorus. So while they are delicious, they are also helping repair cells and build red blood cells.

**Onion** binds to food for faster breakdown and more efficient absorption.

**Pinoli seeds** (pine nut seeds) are a delicious variation to your nuts for a quick snack.

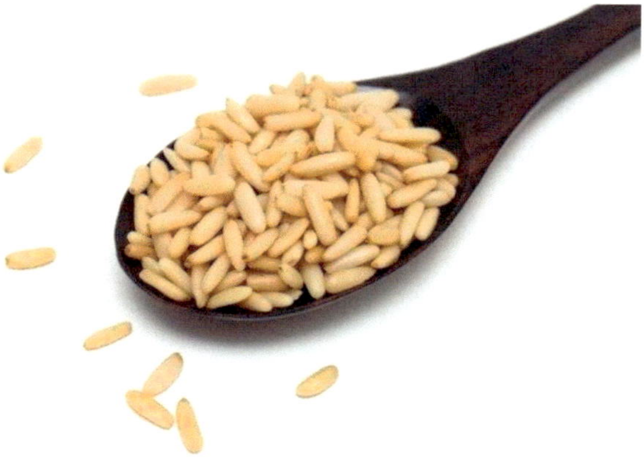

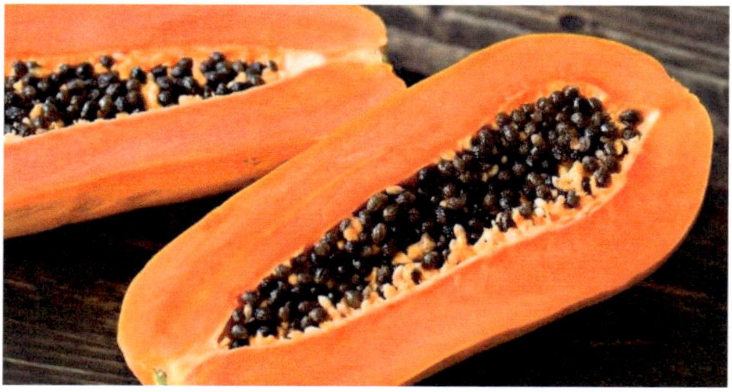

**Papaya** - did you know this helps lower cholesterol and lose weight, plus improves digestion? Try this instead of pineapple for a variation in Doc's Energy Bars.

**Quinoa** is a grain-like seed that has impressed lots of nutritionists with its ability to act as both a protein and a fiber that aids in weight loss. Did you know that quinoa is an ideal source of manganese, phosphorus, and magnesium?

**Radishes** helps strengthen the immune system, lowers blood pressure, and is a good fiber.

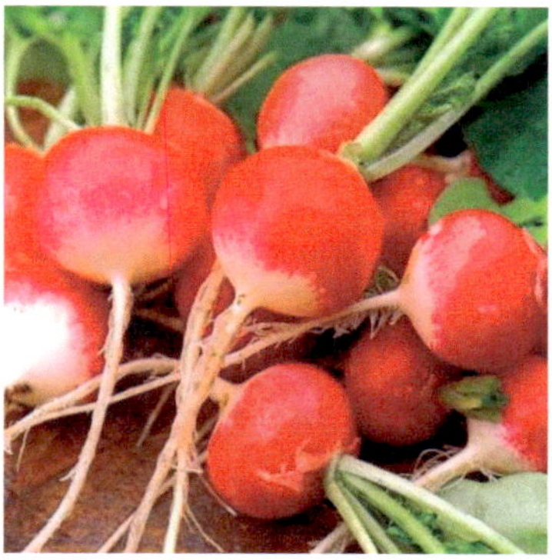

**Saffron** is a magical spice that can both help manage blood sugar (manganese) and act as a natural anti-depressant.  It has also been shown beneficial in increasing bone mass density.  What soup spice could be more magical?

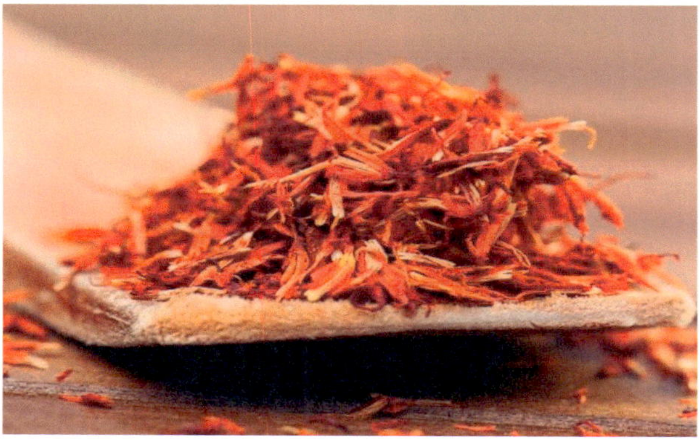

**Stevia** (herb) was shown to be over 200 times sweeter than sugar! It comes from a green-leaf plant in South America but be cautious. Several "Stevia sweeteners" actually have many other ingredients … including cane sugar. (Read the label.) Dozens of clinical research studies have shown stevia's ability to help reduce obesity and cancer.

**Tarragon** is a delicious spice (try on lamb) that also helps neutralize free radicals. It has high levels of potassium, which are good for your heart muscle and help to reduce artery clogging plaque.

(When I asked my boy to name a food starting with "U," he proudly announced, "Upside down cake!")

**Umeboshi** is similar to an apricot in the sour, salty taste, and is very beneficial in reducing nausea. In a recent Japanese study of 1303 subjects, it was proven significantly beneficial in reducing GERD symptoms.

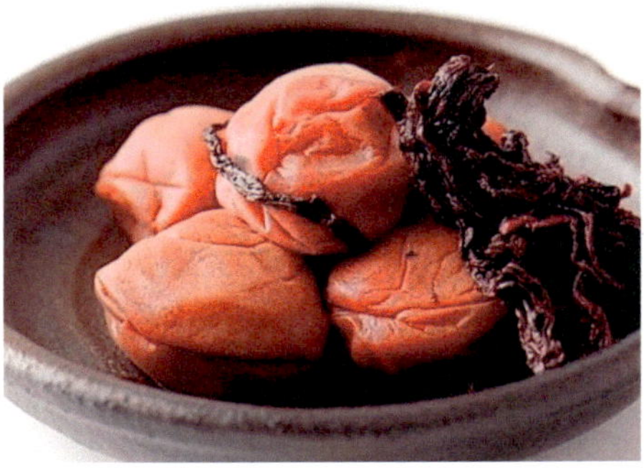

**Vanilla** actually comes from orchids native to Central America. Did you know that vanilla is both an antioxidant and also used as an antibacterial, shown beneficial in reducing staph infections? What if it could reduce depression and colorectal cancer? (This is why you should read the articles from my reference list.)

**Wasabi** is a Japanese horseradish and we're back to heating up the metabolism. It is great with sushi and dense vegetables. (Remember, don't cook the color out of food; this is a sign you're leaving nutrients behind!)

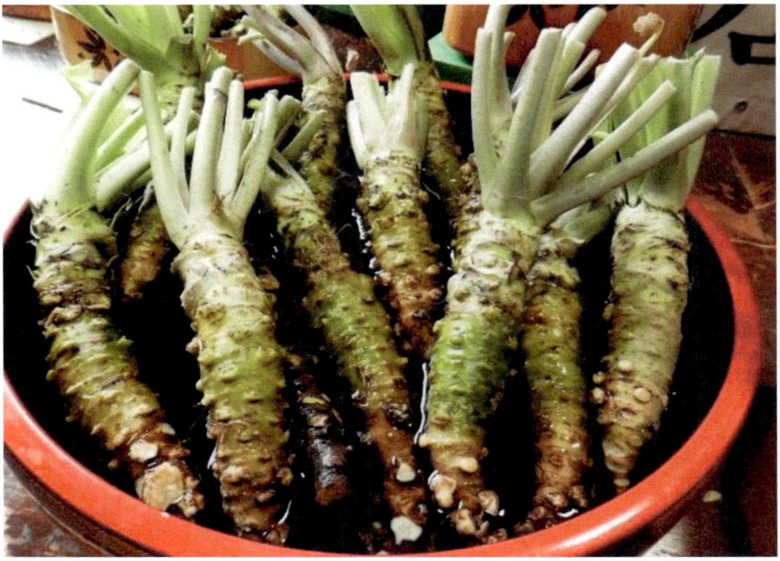

**Walnuts** are the most nutrient dense nut that can also be ground down into a powder.

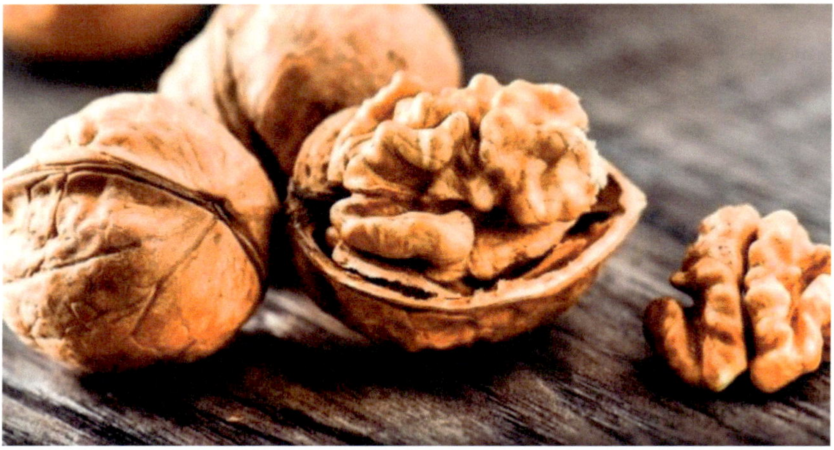

**Ximenia** is a fruit that repotebly has amazing healing properties for the skin. The seeds are dense in oil (67%) which is moisturizing to the skin when applied topically. It also has abundant antibacterial, anti-viral, and antifungal properties.

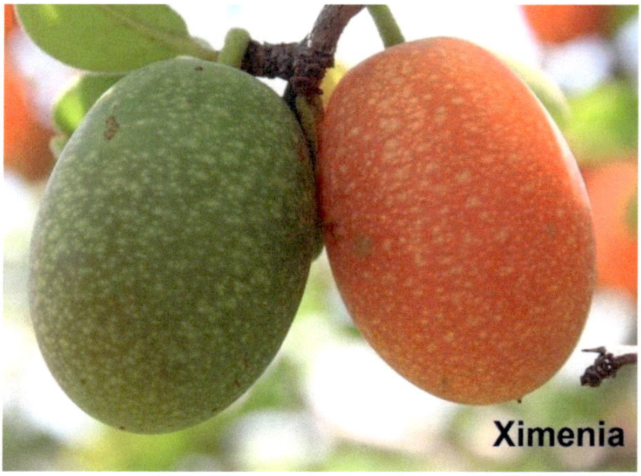

**Xigua** is a sweet yellow melon similar to what we call "watermelon." It has a unique property of cleansing the kidneys and like watermelon, can also act as a diuretic to reduce blood pressure!

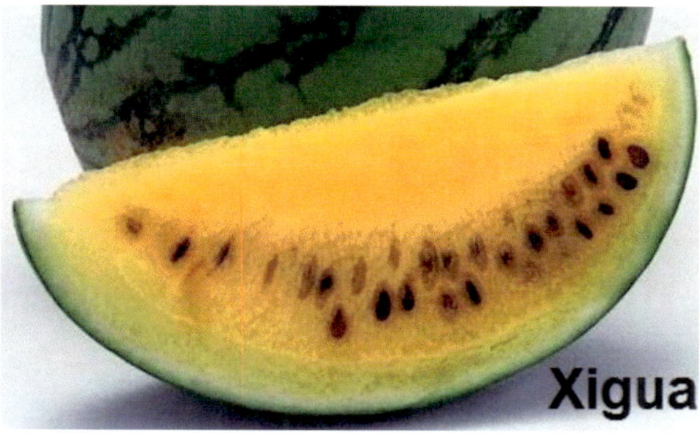


**Zucchini** surprises many in its ability to aid in weight loss. This is due to the dense fiber in zucchini (which is similar to the indigestible fiber in prebiotics). Zucchini is made up of water and polysaccharides.

The polysaccharides (complex carbohydrates) are particularly good for the heart since they reduce inflammation.

***Digest this:*** "The more you talk about negative things in your life, the more you call them in. Speak victory not defeat!" – Pastor Joel Osteen (Lakewood Church Houston)

# CHAPTER 7
# Holistic Wellness
## Taste of Victory: Beer belly traded for a Flat Stomach

Mike never had a problem with a slow metabolism in college; we were teammates on the rugby team at Texas State University (Renegade Rugby!). However, after graduating, Mike quickly gained a beer belly, which affected the position he played since he was getting heavy and could not run as fast. After consulting with me, he realized he was not eating often enough. He only ate two hamburgers, once a day.

He used PAN-5, particularly the Aerobic-surge, for 2 months and lost 20 pounds, and his body became more dense. In a few more months, Mike had a six-pack to flash after the "old boys" had victory over a young college rugby team at a tournament.

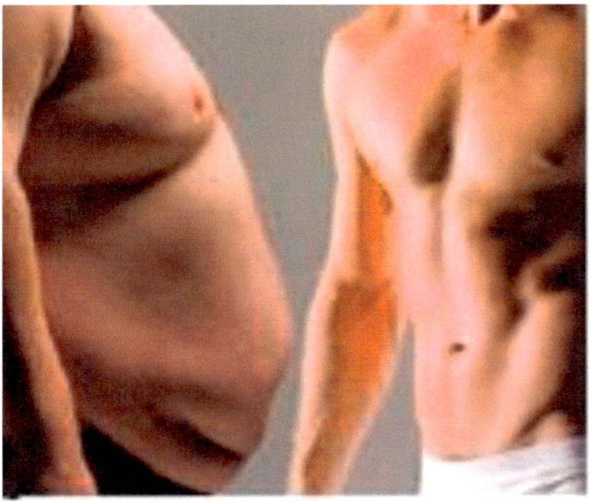

## PAN-5

Again, the formula for wellness is PAN-5. "P" stands for eating single **Portion-size meals** or snacks (less than two cups, five times per day). This is a portion size you could consume in two minutes if necessary. Eating more slowly has been shown to increase metabolic rates, but this is a functional description of the size of a single portion or, eaten every two to three hours. "A" stands for the **Aerobic-surge exercises** (75% of maximum heart rate) for 2 minutes, 5 times per day, and "N" for **Natural foods**, which should be eaten five times per day. (Think of natural as a raw food.)

Research has shown that eating smaller portion sizes also burns more fat. The FDA and Center for Disease Control (CDC) teamed up to sponsor a broad investigation of "Portion Sizes: Now and Then." The bottom line is that the western world's average portion size has increased substantially in the past two decades. One book and several studies may give the right template for the "correct" portion size.

In *The Metabolism Advantage* (2006), Dr. Berardi recommends eating every two to three hours. His book states, "Each time you eat, you stimulate your metabolism for a short period of time, which means that the more often you eat, the more you'll increase your metabolism. *Eating every 2 to 3 hours feeds muscle and starves fat.* By eating frequently, you reassure your body that you aren't going to starve; that food will always be available. Skipping breakfast, eating only a sandwich for lunch, and pigging out at dinner, on the other hand, frightens your body into storing fat, just in case your next meal never comes."

Dr. Dan Benardot's research at Georgia State University clearly showed that the more frequent eating patterns yielded lower body fat and higher muscle mass. In a study he said that eating small, frequent meals and consuming fluid at regular intervals is optimal. Dr. Benardot's research has shown energy deficits from peak and valley meal plans (i.e. eating three times a day with five hours between meals), and such diets showed the highest body fat percentages.

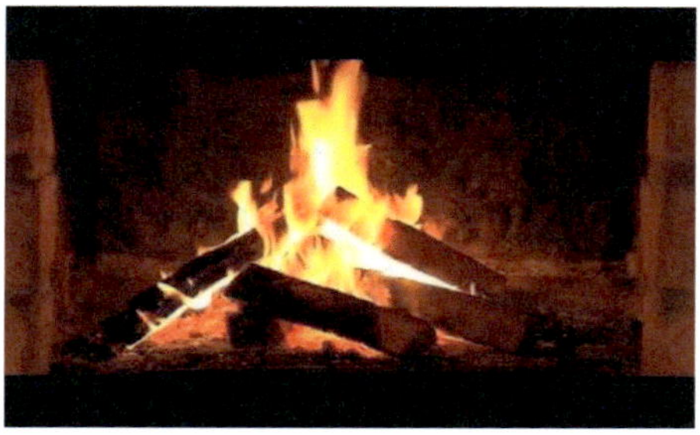

**Think of the portion-size component as a wood-burning fire.** Picture yourself alone in the cold mountains with only a cubic meter stack of wood and kindling to burn for 24 hours. Will you burn it all at once? Of course not; you will slowly “feed the fire” with small additions of wood throughout the day.

If you burned too much wood at once, it would also generate greater quantities of ash, which would not be completely consumed by the fire. So “feeding the fire” of your metabolism keeps the slow fire burning to continually burn the fat.

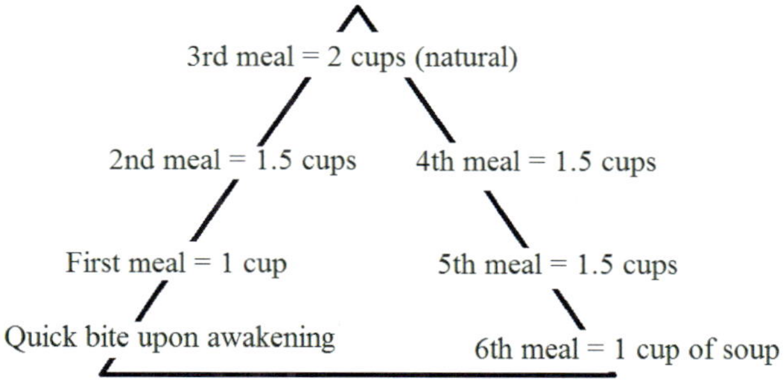


Pyramid meals increase the quantity of foods we eat until our third of five being the largest, before we continually reduce the volume of food we are eating. That is a sequence of meals every two to three hours, which equals five meals in the normal day. The “pyramid” aspect can be linked again to the “flame and fuel” analogy.

This is why it is common practice in bodybuilding to start with the smallest, lightest meal and progress until the third meal (the largest), packed with natural nutrients.

Meal sizes then decrease until the last meal (sixth), which is small and light, similar to the first meal.

Interesting studies have looked at changes in portion size and lack of awareness by subjects and consumers. In a laboratory (Dilberti et al 2004), subjects were fed a 50% greater serving of a pasta dish and in a post-meal survey, only 7% of the subjects noted the increased portion size! Portion size has been proclaimed as an integral factor in weight loss, but consumers may not be conscious of the appropriate volumes of food. While some restaurants admit that they consciously feed patrons more than appropriate volumes of food, 69% of customers report that they regularly eat all of the food served. That is interesting because almost 73% of the US population is overweight. Does being taught to "clean our plate" affect our pattern of eating as adults?

Again research has shown that one should eat a larger total volume of food but in smaller, more numerous doses. Dr. Rolls' systematic review (Rolls 2002) study stated that when large portions are available, people continue to eat more. Think of the fuel analogy; people are taking on more fuel than they need that if not consumed, will be "stored" as fat.

**Consuming single portion-sized meals was further proven by Dr. Foster and colleagues from**

**Temple University** in a study of 69 obese patients with type II diabetes (2009). The subjects were categorized as "obese" because they had a BMI ≥ 39. The subjects' mean age was 52 years and half of the population were African American. One group consumed only portion-sized meals (four times a day) for three months and the other group only received education with no control over the portion sizes of food.

After three months, there was a significant difference in all variables:

- Weight decreased for the portion-size group by 8.2 kg (18 lbs.) vs 0 kg for the education group.
- Waist circumference was reduced 7.6 cm (3.3 inches) for the portion-size group vs. 0 cm for the education group.
- Blood pressure was lowered in the portion-size group.
- HbA1c (average blood glucose over time) was reduced in the portion-size group.
- Systolic blood pressure was reduced for portion-size group.
- Triglycerides and total cholesterol were reduced for the portion-size group.

Then the education group was “crossed over” into eating portion-sized meals and they also showed a subsequent change in weight, waist circumference, etc. Eating single portion-sized meals reduces weight and waistline, and improves one’s health.

## Natural Remedies

There are natural remedies that can be used in conjunction with pharmaceutical treatments *after* your thyroid and testosterone levels are optimal. You can see if these natural treatments can either reduce the pharmacological treatments or replace them. (This is integrative medicine when using both traditional, allopathic medicine plus holistic medicine.)

Testosterone studies have shown that when raising a person’s heart rate with vigorous resistance exercise (like your **Aerobic- surge**), it increases testosterone levels. The “top 10” natural treatments to increase testosterone are as follows:

- **Reduce Obesity**
- **Increase Zinc** (However, take less than 40 mg of zinc/day.)
- **Eliminate Alcohol Consumption** (One study showed a 7% raise in testosterone after eliminating alcohol.)

- **Reduce Stress**
- **Increase Exercise Intensity** (l2-minute, aerobic surges)
- **Eliminate Sugar**
- **Sleep More**
- **Eat Healthy Fats** (like avocado, olive oil, coconut oil, tuna)

**Maca** (*lepidium meyenii*) from the mountains of Peru, has shown effective in raising sexual function and reducing erectile dysfunction in a randomized controlled (animal trial) by Zheng et al (2000). After 22-days, it raised testosterone levels.

**What about Thyroid deficiencies?** Natural remedies for thyroid secretion include flaxseed and fish oils. Here are other natural remedies for hypothyroid secretion:

- **Iodine** is beneficial in increasing thyroid production because it is a building block for both T3 and T4 (The dosage is 150-300 mcg/day.).
- **Selenium** is an integral component of T3, which is the most active thyroid hormone. It is also an effective antioxidant.

- **L-tyrosine** is an amino acid used in the synthesis of T3 production and actually L-tyrosine molecule, with four iodine molecules, is the structure of the T4 thyroid hormone.

***Digest this:*** How often did we run to the swings and eat snacks when we were five or six years old? What was our health then compared to now? Daily medications now?

# CHAPTER 8

## Natural Fuel

**Taste of Victory:** "Bill" always tried to get to the gym and eat the right foods, but his erratic schedule and "work lunches" had contributed to his overweight, sedentary state. He started using the energy surge exercise bout when he first awoke and later read devotions while riding the recumbent bicycle at the YMCA. He felt good about what he was doing! When he had meals at restaurants, he would limit his choice to use portion size as his variable, and would often order a small hamburger without fries to elevate his metabolism. He would always estimate how much of the plate's serving would fit into a cereal bowl (two minutes of casual eating).

Bill felt empowered by this and while he only needed to lose 20 pounds, he decreased his blood pressure from 160/80 to 125/75 (20%). After four more months, he was taken off his medicine for high cholesterol.

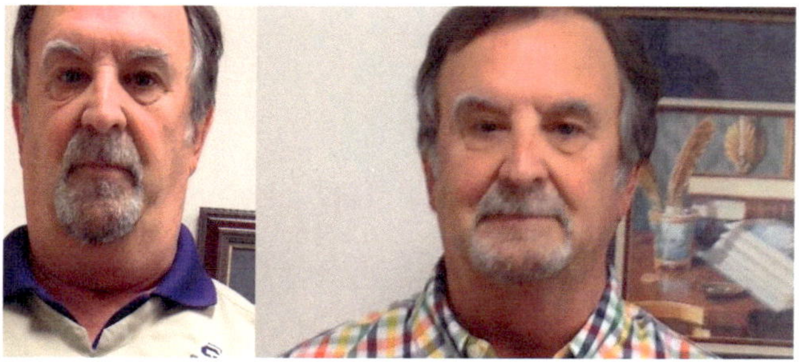

**Our Pastor lost 20lbs and 20" in Two Months!**

**The "fuel" (food) we take into our bodies determines how and what will be consumed as energy, and is either used for building new cellular structures or stored as fat.** "Natural nutrition" means consuming products that are or were first raw and have not been processed or modified. Ask yourself, "Did God put this on the planet?" Organic foods are the ideal ingredients in your Rightsize program, but cost and availability often impairs the choice of organic foods. **However, eating fresh, unprocessed foods will be equally beneficial for your initial RightSize program.**

It is easy to think of eating raw fruits and vegetables or cooking foods without processed ingredients, but we must also understand the functions of the seven nutrients and the metabolism of fats and sugars. This chapter will provide you with recommendations for planning the right fuel types (think of it as octane) and the right volume (how often you should fill up). What are your molecular needs?

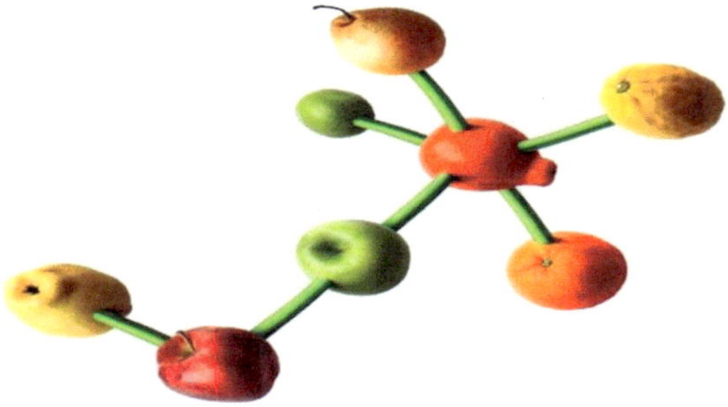

## Nutrients

The six essential nutrients that our bodies need to operate are:

- **Carbohydrates**, used as immediate fuel
- **Fats**, needed for cell walls (epithelium) and organ insulation. This can also act as fuel when training in the aerobic threshold.
- **Proteins**, to provide the structural framework that our bodies continually need
- **Fiber**, to assist in the digestion process
- **Vitamins**, involved in chemical regulation. For example, vitamin D increases calcium absorption.
- **Water**, needed for nearly all bodily functions, as well as transporting nutrients throughout the body. Water is needed in reactions to break down fats but too much causes hyponatremia (lost sodium and other elements).

Now that you have a basic understanding of each nutrient, let's take a deeper dive!

**Dietary carbohydrates** are substances containing carbon, hydrogen, and oxygen. These substances can be broken down into sugars (glucose). The function of the carbohydrate is to provide energy for cellular work, maintain cell structure, generate heat, regulate fat, and assist in protein metabolism. The type of carbohydrate is determined by the heat generated through metabolism of these nutrients. A calorie is the heat required (or generated) to increase one gram of water by one degree, Celsius. The calories needed for optimal functioning are estimated to be 2,000 per day.

I don't necessarily want you to "count calories," but here's some perspective: while the average calories needed per day is around 2,000 with normal activity, the average American consumes an estimated 3,900 calories per day. If we are eating the wrong processed foods, our metabolism and needed calories will go down and any fuel not needed will be stored as fat. It has been shown that every two decades, average consumption has increased by 700 calories. This means that in the next twenty years our population of obese and overweight people will rise. How much did Americans eat in the

1920s? How fat were they? (In the 1920s, the obesity rate was under 8% compared to today's rate of almost 40%!) Remember grandmother saying, "You are what you eat?"

**Simple carbohydrates** (carbs) are the mono-saccharides and di-saccharides formed by simple sugar molecules that have little nutritive value. Examples of simple carbohydrates include glucose, fructose, galactose, or combinations of those sugars. An apple is a simple carbohydrate.

**Complex carbohydrates** are the valuable fuels which boast three or more sugar molecules linked together, such as starches, dextrins, and glycogen. Complex carbs such as grains or seeds also include dietary fibers which are actually not "digested," but used to process digestion of other food stuffs. These are plant products. The next variable in carbohydrates is whether they are soluble or not.

"Solubility" is the property which allows a particle to be dissolved into a liquid or gas. Sugar is soluble because it can fully dissolve into water, but fiber is not. Variables that affect a component's solubility are heat (temperature), volume, pressure, molecular polarity (how fast can the molecules be removed to "mix"), and the rate or speed of solution. So if a substance is easily soluble, then it will require low energy for breakdown and will therefore be consumed easily without requiring high energy or work for breakdown, like sugar in water. But substances that are insoluble require greater energy for breakdown, like fiber or fat.

**Dietary fats,** or **lipids,** are necessary and have multiple complex roles in a body's function. Fats are a required component of the cell linings, so fats are integral for cell structure and integrity. Fats are needed to protect the organs and can be thought of as "shock absorbers," and are also vital for carrying vitamins A, D, E, and K. On the contrary, excessive ingestion of fats can lead to a "fatty heart," in which case it will keep a body from functioning optimally. The heart muscles are made to contract and pump blood but, since fat cannot contract, it impairs the muscular contraction.

**Fats can be used for fuel**, but in order for that to happen, aerobic exercise is required. This is because the maximum oxygen intake is required to break down fats. Think of long endurance athletes who train for marathons, century bicycle rides (100 miles), or endurance swimmers. These athletes have low body fat because their continual, prolonged exercise in the Aerobic Threshold consumes fat as the primary fuel. Saturated fatty acids are long molecular chains that are difficult to break apart. That is why saturated fatty acids are carried as molecules through the blood and can clog arteries (arthrosclerosis).

**Dietary proteins** are complex organic compounds with the same elements as in sugars, but proteins also contain nitrogen and amino acids. Sugars are often circular structures and fat molecules have long single-chain structures, but the molecular structure of protein is often a “ball” of amino acid chains, which boast the greatest structure (See Figure 3.).

**Figure 3.**

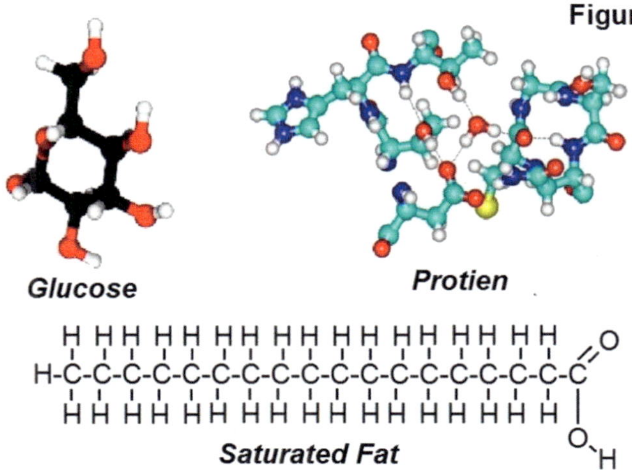


The function of protein includes building structures including bones, muscles, internal organs, hair, nails and skin. Proteins also repair such structures and form active molecules such as enzymes for initiating reactions via hormones and antibodies. These structures are also important for the normal balance of body fluids. These can be broken down as an energy source. This is why a healthy diet with protein is important, so that the body is not breaking down muscle as fuel while fats are being stored. The old adage “muscle turns into fat” is wrong, but muscle atrophy (decrease in size and strength) often occurs simultaneously to fat expansion.

The types of proteins are differentiated by the type and number of amino acids. The 20 amino acids are “building blocks.” Nine amino acids are “essential” because your body cannot produce them. The body does not store amino acids, so these essential amino acids must be ingested every day. One then may question, which protein is the most complete? The answer is “the egg.” The egg contains all 20 amino acids. While the egg contains all amino acids, it is interesting that only about 10% of a full egg is actually protein.

| **Essential** | **Nonessential** |
|---|---|
| histidine | alanine |
| isoleucine | arginine |
| leucine | aspartic acid |
| lysine | cysteine |
| methionine | glutamic acid |
| phenylalanine | glutamine |
| threonine | glycine |
| tryptophan | proline |
| valine | serine |
| | tyrosine |
| | asparagine |
| | selenocysteine |

**Vitamins** facilitate chemical reactions; however, vitamins provide no energy.  Vitamins exist in both water and fat soluble types.  The purpose of vitamins is to promote growth and stability in life stages ranging from pregnancy to reducing osteoporosis in the elderly stage. Some vitamins also serve as antioxidants, which help reduce the cascade of erroneous cell replication that could become cancerous.

The primary vitamins, functions, and food sources are listed in the table below.

| VITAMIN | FUNCTION | FOOD SOURCES |
| --- | --- | --- |
| Vitamin A | Renews eyes & skin | Liver, Milk, Cheese |
| Vitamin B1 | Energy absorption | Whole grains |
| Vitamin B2 | Energy production | Poultry, beef, liver, eggs |
| Vitamin B3 | Use Fat for Energy | Mushroom, fish, poultry |
| Vitamin B6 | Produce Glycogen | Banana, Potato |
| Vitamin B12 | Produce DNA struc. | Milk, rice, soy |
| Biotin | Protien to carbs | Sweet potatoes |
| Vitamin C | Prevent Cell Damage | Citrus fruit, cabbage, brocoli |
| Vitamin D | Transport Calcium | Dairy products, eggs, fish |
| Vitamin E | Cell structure | Yellow and green vegetables |
| Vitamin E | ↓↓ Arteriosclerosis | oatmeal, wheatgerm, almond |
| Vitamin E | ↑↑ Immune system | Avocados, leafy green veg. |
| Folate | DNA structure | Beets, brocoli, peas, oranges |
| Iron | Oxygen transport | Peas, egg yolk, fish |
| Vitamin K | Create protiens | Collards, kale, spinach, soy |
| Vitamin K | Clots bleeding | above, plus brocoli, |

**Minerals** are indestructible, inorganic structures listed on the chemical periodic table. The macro minerals include calcium, chloride, magnesium, phosphorus, potassium, sulfur, and sodium. Again water is the most important nutrient, particularly for all chemical reactions in your body, including breaking down fats. Examples of minerals in our diet include calcium from milk and copper from seafood or nuts.

The true bottom line of why optimal, natural nutrition is important can be understood with the fuel and fire analogy of one's metabolism. When a small flame is doused with a quickly consumable fuel (like gasoline), the flame bursts high but quickly dies out. When swallowing a tablespoon of sugar, it will burn quickly. However, placing a slow burning fuel on the fire will help to increase the flame and continue burning at an elevated rate. In a similar manner, eating whole, unprocessed foods that are full of the optimal nutrients (like almonds) will help to maintain an elevated basal metabolic rate.

**Antioxidants** are important for preventing disease. Here are the top foods containing antioxidants, proven in medical research:

**Blackberries**
**Walnuts (best nut)**
**Strawberries**
**Antichoke hearts**
**Cranberries**
**Rasberries**
**Pecans**
**Blueberries**
**Ground clover**
**Dark Grapes**
**Dark Veggies (broccoli)**
**Sweet Potatoes**
**Green Tea**

For optimal nutrition and balance, one can access the current FDA website, www.ChooseMyPlate.gov. This is a tremendous resource and has information on dishes, nutrient tracking, calorie calculations, eating tips (even for vegetarians eating out), and much more. This website was used successfully by subjects in a study led by Dr. Willis and Dr. Smith in 2012. The old food pyramid, www.FoodPyramid.com, also has volumes of delicious, healthy recipes.

One benefit of natural foods is that they trigger the metabolic feedback of being satiated. This means your body will tell you when you are full compared to several noted "weight loss" foods, "low calorie" ingredients, or fatty carbohydrates (chips) that do not give your body such feedback.

When eating natural foods, remember to avoid processed toppings, dressings, or sauces. If you use anything packaged (from salad dressing to mac n cheese), make sure it is *organic*!

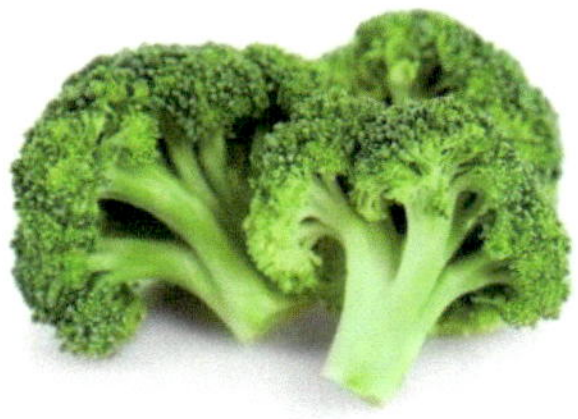

## Here are foods that accelerate fat loss:

| |
|---|
| **Asparagus** (increases folic acid and glutathione) |
| **Apricots** (increase vitamin A, C, fiber, iron, and calcium) |
| **Apples** (increases peristalsis, detoxification, and better digestion) |
| **Beets** (bind to fats, decrease water retention, and reduce colon cancer) |
| **Carrots** (provide beta-carotene and bind to cholesterol) |
| **Chili Peppers** (increase metabolism ~ *Burn baby burn!*) |
| **Cucumber** (act as a natural diuretic and increase metabolism) |
| **Garlic** (acts as a diuretic and increases metabolism with antibiotic effects) |
| **Grapefruit** (increases the metabolism and is proven to aid in fat loss) |
| **Green Tea** (increases oxidation for increased fat breakdown) |
| **Onion** (binds to food for faster breakdown) |

***Digest this:*** Remember to forecast your food for the outcomes you desire! Forecast Victory … and it is yours! (Mark 11:24)

## SECTION III

## CHAPTER 9 Recipes to Success

**Taste of Victory**: "CJ" lost her first child in delivery and soon became pregnant again. After delivery of her healthy, beautiful son, she was hurt when she retained weight and people asked, "Are you pregnant again?" She began adding an Aerobic-surge, quick-walk to her daily routine.

People often ask, "If you use only one of Doc's protocols, will it work?" CJ's answer is *"Yes!"* The energy surge worked so well that she is now a professional model and can be seen in many of fitness and stretching photos! You have seen more of her photos throughout this book.

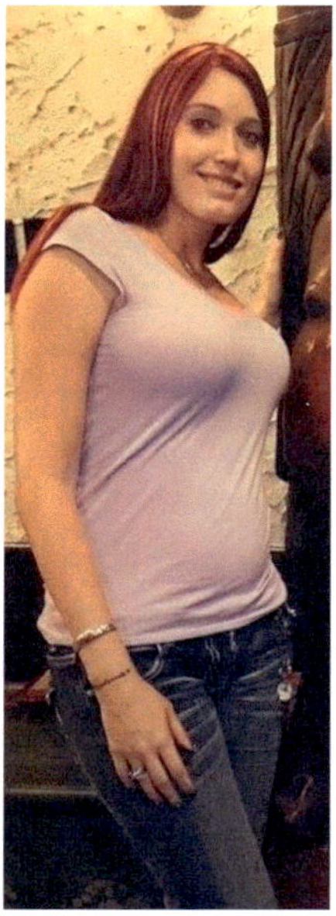

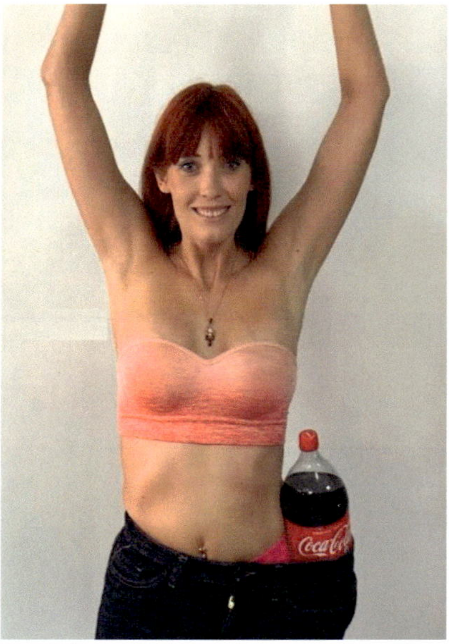

**The recipes to** success are listed in alphabetical order and thanks Mom for all of the teaching and summer jobs at Mom & Miss Judy's Secret Hostesses catering company!

## Annie's Sautéed Pork and Potatoes

1) Chop up 4 pork tenderloins and stir fry in olive oil for less than 5 minutes with black pepper, salt, and ½ red onion.
2) Throw 2 cups of shredded red potato into the same oil. At the last minute, toss in strips of cucumber skins and cook just enough to soften.
3) Serve with steamed rice and enjoy!

*Bon Appétit!*

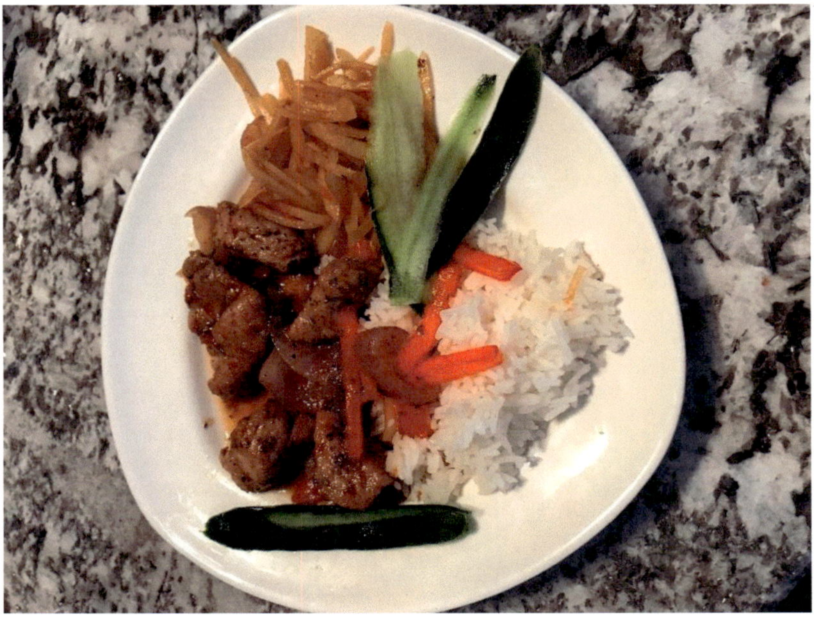

## Bar B Que Sauce

1 tbsp butter
1 small onion, diced
3 cloves roasted garlic
1 large sweet potato, cut into ½" slivers
½ c apple cider
1 small (3 oz.) can organic tomato paste
1 tsp paprika
1 tsp salt
½ tsp chipotle powder
1 tbsp apple cider vinegar

Heat the butter in a medium skillet on medium. Add the onions and cook until brown and caramelized (15 min). At the same time, cook the sweet potatoes and apple cider in a medium pot with just enough water to cover the sweet potatoes. Bring to a boil and then simmer for only 15 minutes. Strain and remove liquid from the pot. Combine the sautéed onions and potatoes in a food processor before adding the other ingredients. Blend until the consistency is like that of ketchup.

*Bon Appétit!*

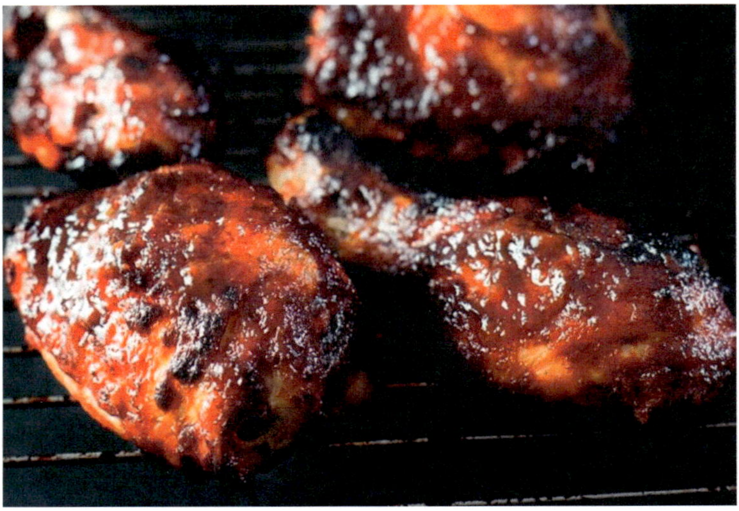

## Beach Bean Peppers

Combine these ingredients in a large mixing bowl:

1 red bell pepper, chopped

1 yellow bell pepper, chopped

1 large fresh jalapeño with seeds removed, chopped

1/2 red onion

Mix all of these ingredients in the large mixing bowl.

Steam two cups fresh green beans for six minutes. Cover the mixed peppers with the hot green beans. The hot beans will soften the peppers and onions without removing the colors or nutrients. Mix together and cover with a light glaze of ½ cup organic balsamic vinaigrette! *Bon Appétit!*

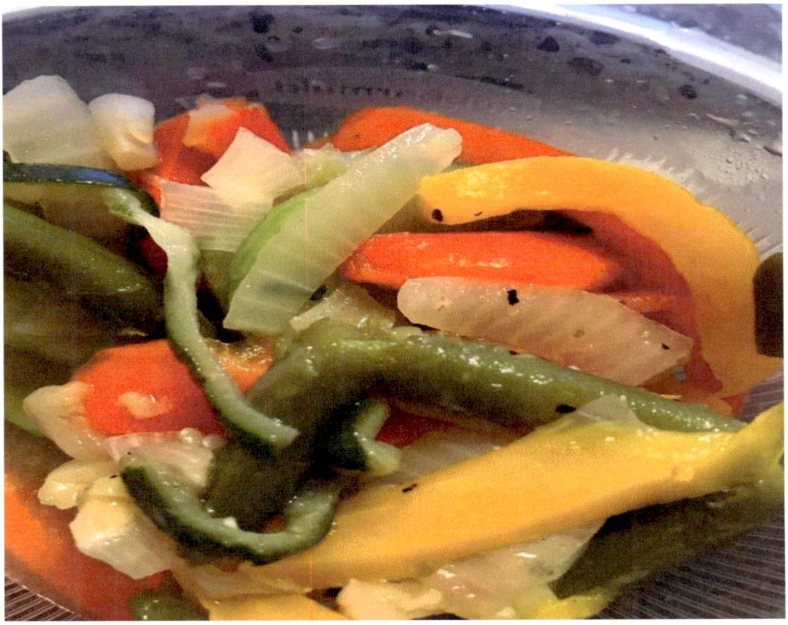

## Blueberry Sweet Bread

2 cups organic flour 1 ½ tsp baking powder
½ tsp salt
½ c whipping cream
½ stick butter
1 c blueberries

1 c brown sugar
2/3 c vanilla yogurt

2 tsp cinnamon
2 eggs, beaten
1 ½ tsp baking soda

Combine dry ingredients in a bowl. Cut in butter with a pastry blender until the mixture resembles coarse meal. Add blueberries and toss well. Add yogurt and egg whites, stirring just until the dry ingredients are moistened and dough is sticky.

Place in 6x6" loaf pan or mini pans. Bake at 350° for 35 minutes or until the loaf rises and gets firm. Cool for 30 minutes before slicing.

*Bon Appétit!*

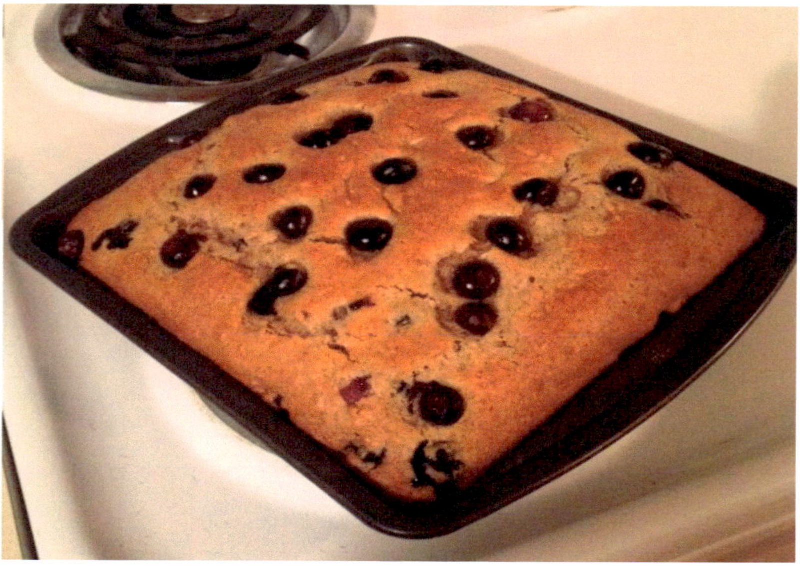

# Braised Trout

<u>Ingredients:</u>
4 fresh 6" trout filets
Italian spices (allspice, basil, sage, garlic,thyme, rosemary (change for allergies)
1 lime sectioned

<u>Directions</u>: lightly glaze a large skillet with extra virgin olive oil and then heat on Medium-high for a few minutes (not as hot as blackening).

- Squeeze lime juice on each of the filets (1/4 lime slice for each) and then gently sprinkle on the dry italian seasoning mix.
- Place filets (spice side down) in the skillet
- Cook for just a few (3) minutes and then spray lime juice on naked side before gently sprinkling spices and flip so the new spice side cooks for another 3-4 minutes. (They will already be flaking apart!) *Bon Appétit!*

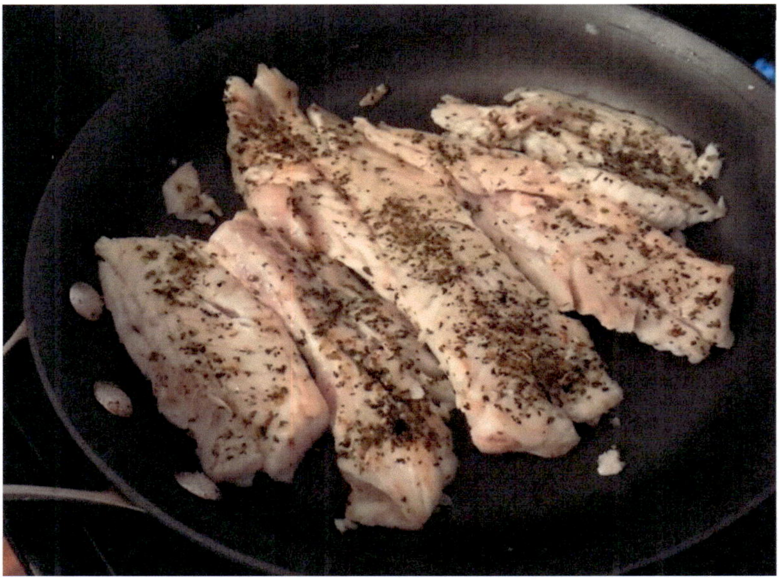

# Cabbage-Garlic Stir Fry

(Try it before raining your nose and enjoy the options!)
½ head cabbage (or kale)
½ cup Endives or leeks
½ clove crushed garlic or 1 table curry (That is out of the JacknBox!)

Simply stir fry quickly and you can exchange almost anything! Ever throught why only 5% of Chinese people are obese compared to almost 40% in the USA, UK, etc.?

*Bon Appétit!*

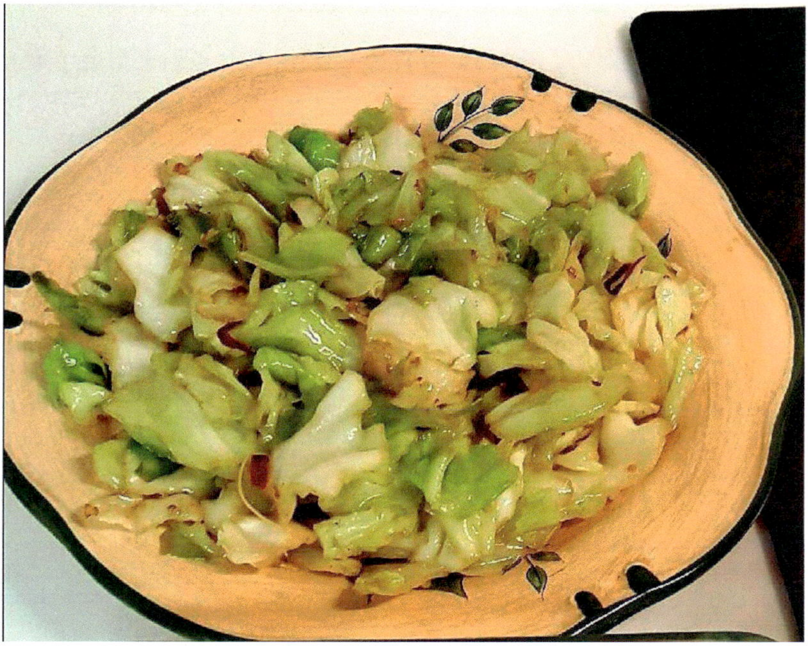

# Caribbean Wings

6 lbs. chicken wings
1 habanero, seeded and chopped
1/4 c soy sauce
1/4 c honey
1/4 c brown sugar
2 tbsp sugar
2 tsp fennel seed
2 tsp Cayenne Pepper
2 tsp allspice
2 tsp dried thyme
1 tsp ground ginger
4 garlic cloves, chopped
4 green onions, chopped
1/4 c apple cider vinegar
1/4 c lime juice
1/4 c orange juice

Combine all ingredients (except wings) in a food processor and blend until smooth. Remove 1 cup to use for a basting sauce. Place chicken wings into a large zip lock bag(s) and pour remaining marinade over them. Squeeze, flip and make sure that all of the wings are coated before you refrigerate 4 to 6 hours. Preheat oven to 350 degrees. Line 2 sheet trays with parchment paper. Remove chicken from bag, place on the baking sheets, and bake 20 minutes. Boil the 1 cup sauce that you saved for basting and then reduce heat to 30% as you let it thicken. After 20 minutes, remove chicken from oven, and brush wings with the glaze. Raise the heat to 400 degrees and cook chicken for another 20 minutes.

*Bon Appétit!*

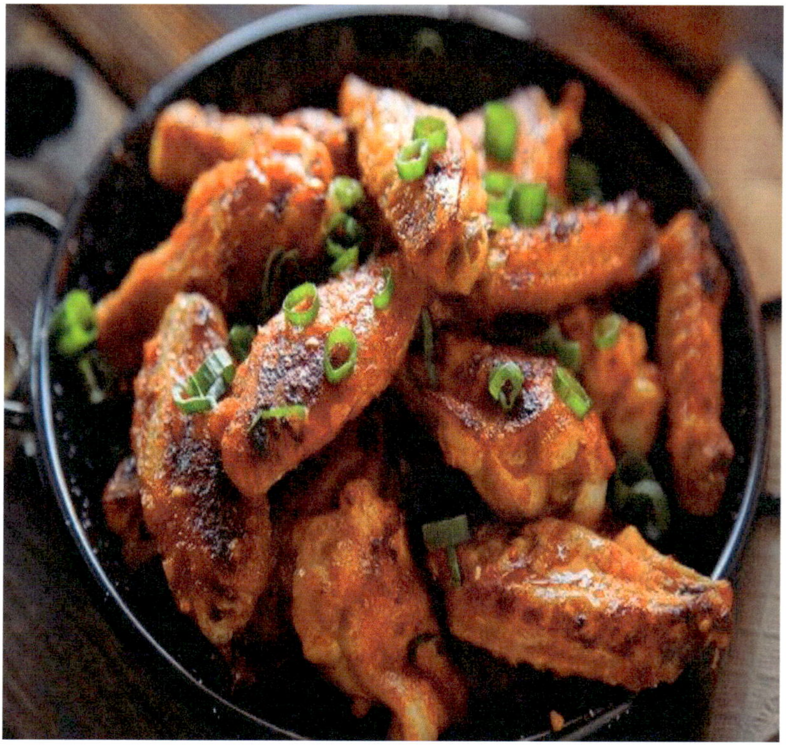

# Chalupa Compuesta

4-6 organic tostadas (or toast natural corn tortillas)
1 can organic pinto beans
¼ red onion
½ c sharp cheddar cheese
2 chicken breasts, cooked in crockpot batch
2-3 ripe avocados
½ c homemade salsa
chopped lettuce
Roma tomatoes

Toast the corn tortillas for just a few minutes and leave in warm toaster or oven to become crispy. Smash the organic beans and add 1 tbsp of salsa. Spread beans on the crisp tortilla and add onions, chicken, and cheese before you toast again for 1-2 minutes. Top with lettuce, tomatoes, avocado (slices or guacamole), and salsa!

*Bon Appétit!*

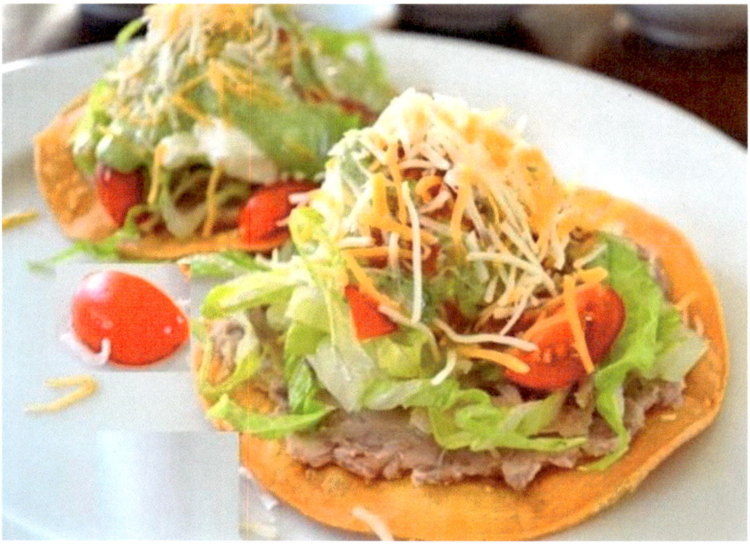

## Chicken Chili

1 tbsp vegetable oil
1 lb. chicken breasts, crockpot cooked
1 onion
2 tbsp chili powder
1 tsp ground cumin
1 tsp ground black pepper
¼ tsp garlic powder
1 ¾ c organic chicken broth
1 c chunky salsa
1 tbsp cane sugar
1 15-oz can organic black beans, dried and rinsed
16 oz. bag of frozen whole kernel corn
1 tsp dried, crushed oregano leaves

One hour before cooking, bring the corn out of the freezer to thaw and chop the onion. Heat the oil in a 4-quart saucepan over medium-high heat. Add the chicken, onion, chili powder, cumin, oregano, black pepper, and garlic powder. Cook until chicken is well browned, stirring frequently to break up meat. Stir the chicken broth, salsa, sugar, beans, and corn into the saucepan. Heat to a boil. Reduce the heat to low.

Cover and cook for 30 minutes. Stir the chili occasionally while cooking.

*Bon Appétit!*

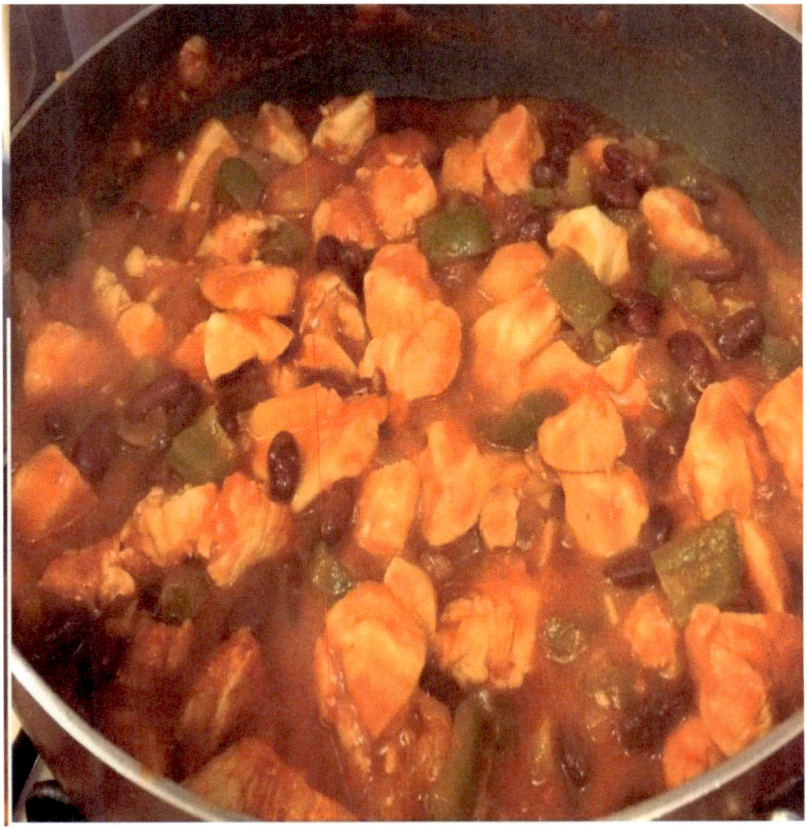

## Chicken Teepee

2 large chicken breasts, preferably already cooked with crockpot recipe
1 c frozen pearl onions
8 button mushrooms, quartered
2 sticks celery, chopped
1/2 c halved baby turnips
Kosher salt
4 c organic chicken broth
1/4 c all-purpose flour
1 tbsp minced parsley
2 tsp minced dill
1/2 tsp finely grated lemon zest
Freshly ground black pepper
2 sheets organic phyllo dough
2 tbsp butter
Paprika

Heat the oil in a large skillet on medium-high heat. Add the carrots, mushrooms, celery, turnips, seasoning, and salt to taste. Cook until the vegetables are light brown, about 8 minutes. Add the onions and cook about 1 minute more. Stir the flour into the vegetables and cook for 1 minute. Pour in the reserved chicken broth and whisk until it comes to a boil.

Reduce the heat slightly and simmer, uncovered, until thick, about 5 to 6 minutes. Stir in the chicken parsley, dill, lemon zest, and pepper, and remove from heat. Now pull out two 6"x6" pans and prepare space for creating your teepees. Butter the bottom of each pan and then set the phyllo into the pan to fill with the shredded chicken and vegetables. Fill and then raise the edges of the dough to seal together as the top of the teepee. (See picture below.) Bake for 10-12 minutes.

*Bon Appétit!*

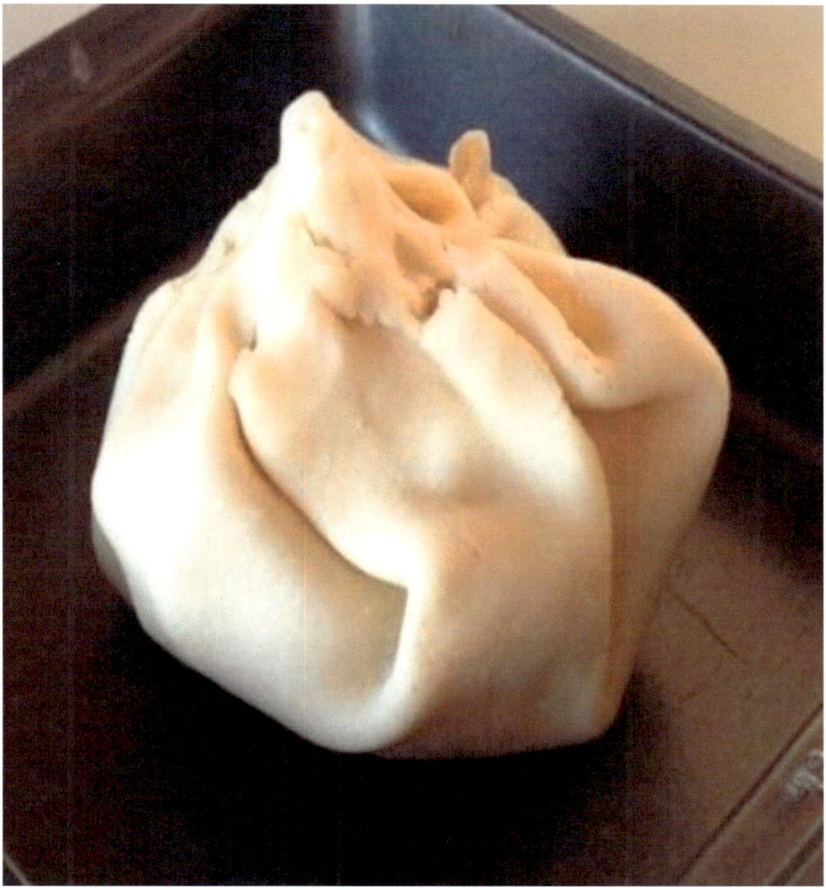

## Chocolate Coconut Bars

Ingredients:
2 cups raw cashews
1.25 cup dried figs (no Sulphur or sugar & cut stems off)
1 cup unsweetened Coconut Flakes (extra for topping)
1 tsp vanilla
2/3 cup or more of dark chocolate or vegan dark chocolate chips to melt
1 tsp cacao powder
Dash sea salt

Directions:

1. Line a square baking pan with parchment paper. Set aside.
2. Place cashew, coconut, salt, vanilla, and figs in food processor. (Blend well = chunks).
3. Pour mixture into baking dish and press down well.
4. While the fig/cashew mix sets in pan, melt your dark chocolate.
5. Melt chocolate in microwave (Pyrex bowl) for 60 seconds, stirring every 30 seconds or on stove top.
6. Pour the chocolate over the cashew/coconut mix and spread evenly.
7. Garnish (top) with coconut or almond slices.
8. Place in freezer for 20 minutes or fridge for a few hrs.
9. Slice into bars and wrap each one in foil for a quick grab and go bar.
10. Best kept in fridge for freshness.

*Bon Appétit!*

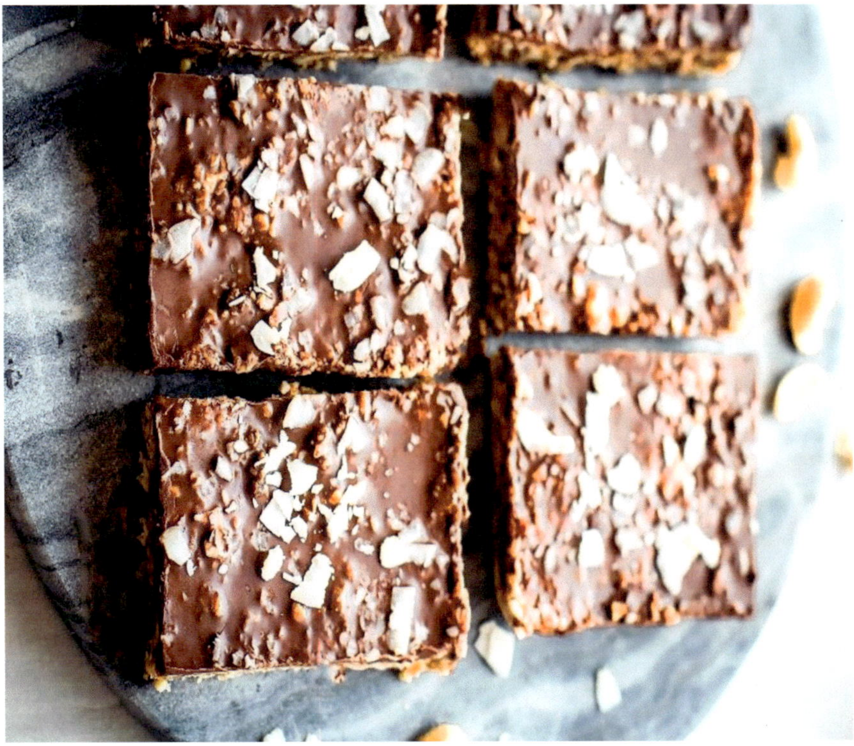

# Crock Pot Lasagna Soup

1 lb. lean ground beef
1 yellow medium yellow onion, diced
3 cloves garlic, finely chopped
1 (28 oz.) can crushed organic tomatoes
1 can (15 oz.) organic tomato sauce
32 oz. organic beef broth
1 tbsp dried basil leaves
1 tbsp dried parsley
½ c water
1 c uncooked organic bowtie pasta
1 chopped zucchini

Salt & pepper to taste

First grill the beef and do not fry meat in a skillet to prevent regenerating the fats. (I normally grill all my meats for the week at one time on Sunday afternoon.) Place the beef and all ingredients (except pasta and zucchini) into the crockpot and cook on low for 7-8 hours. After 7-8 hours, add the uncooked pasta and zucchini for the last 30 minutes of cooking. *Bon Appétit!*

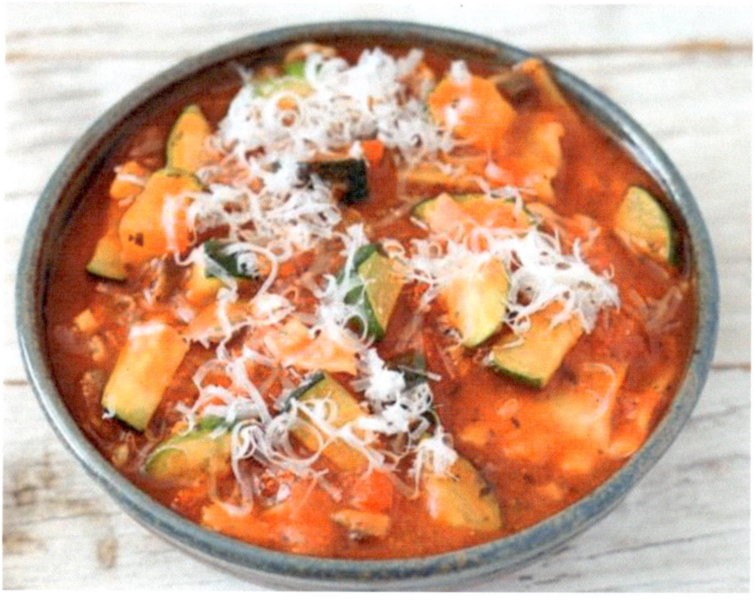

# Doc's Energy Bar

In a large mixing bowl:

- Grind ½ c pecans, then add and grind ½ cup cherries and ½ cup cranberries
  (frozen raw is okay if it contains no added sugars).
- Stir in ½ cup of carob powder.
- Stir in ½ c shredded pineapple (pineapple only, no syrup or sugar).
- Mix in ½ c raw peanut butter (almond butter is better if not allergic)
  (best from the grocery store machine that takes raw peanuts and smashes into peanut butter).
  Mix this vigorously for 2 minutes (with elevated heart rate) for an aerobic surge!

Glaze a 13" Pyrex baking pan with extra virgin olive oil.

Pour in mix (press down) and bake for 60 minutes at 350° (you want it to dry out).

Cover the pan with raw, salted sunflower seeds or sprinkles of Stevia, and cool for 30 minutes.

Garnish with strawberries of other favorite fruit. You can try using raw natural pumpkin as the sticky product and use different fruits and nuts! Send me your recipe with pictures and I'll list this as your variation in the next book.

*Bon Appétit!*

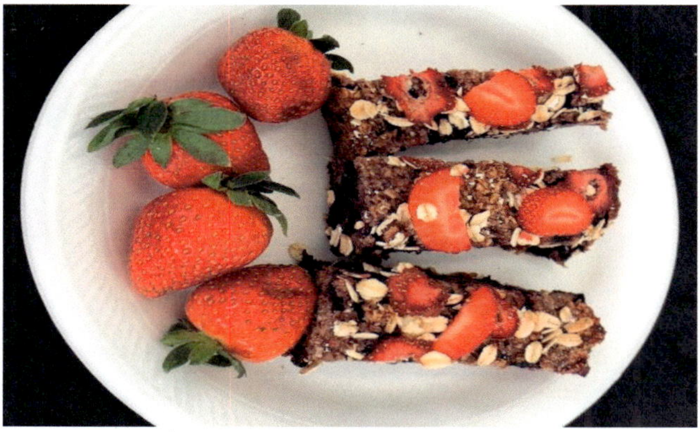

## Doc's Crockpot Chicken

2 lbs chicken (4-6 boneless, skinless chicken breasts)
One bottle organic beer

½ c homemade salsa
1 vrushed raw garlic clove
1 tps Cayenne Pepper
1 tsp ground pepper

Combine all seasoning ingredients plus beer in crockpot. Cook on high for 4 hours, or for 8 hours if your chicken is frozen (all natural), and you have a delicious protein for the next few days!

*Bon Appétit!*

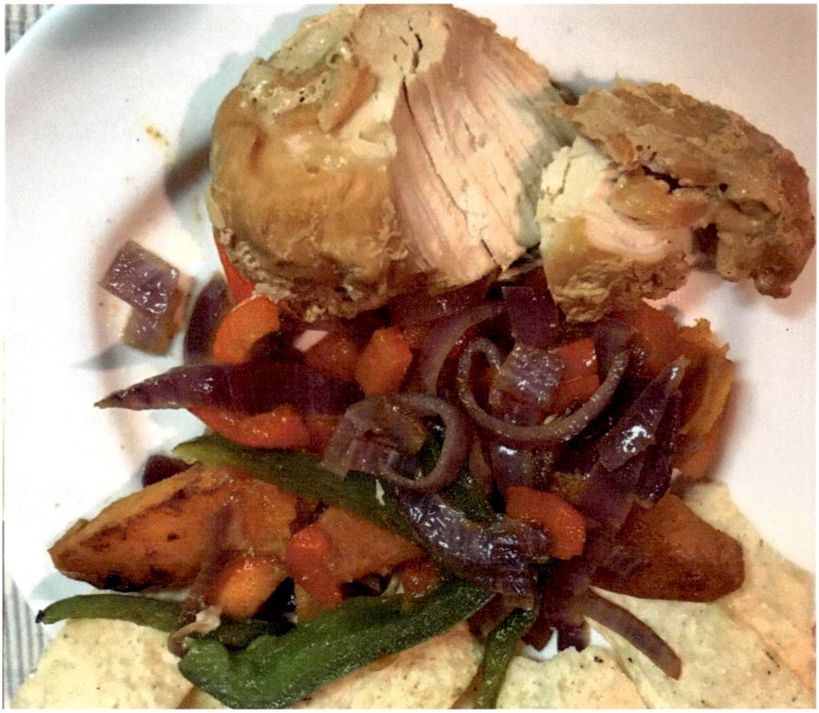

## Fish and Sweet Potatoes

Ingredients:

- 4 fillets of fresh fish, never frozen
- Long (< 6”), thin red yams (Caribbean sweet potatoes), one yam per person
- Fresh cabbage heads, red and green
- Two fresh limes per person
- Ripe avocado, 1/2 per person

Directions:

- Shred/grate the cabbage and squeeze just a small amount of lime on a bowl full of the colorful slaw. Gently toss it once.
- Start the grill on high for 10 minutes.
- Squeeze one half fresh lime on each side of the fish fillets followed by a generous amount of fresh ground black pepper.
- Slice the long, thin yams to 1’ slices and place on the grill with heat reduced to 3/4. (They will cook for 20 minutes total.) Chop if needed.
- Top with island salsa (mango).

*Bon Appétit!*

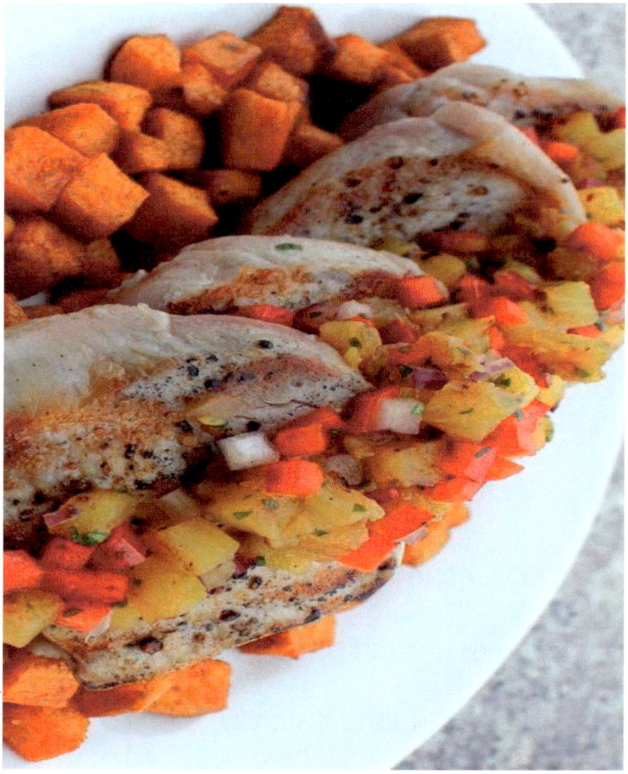

## Fish in Peppers

3 c flaked, cooked lean fish
3 red bell peppers
3 hard-boiled eggs, chopped
3 tbsp sweet pickle relish
½ c diced celery
½ c organic mayo
Parsley
Black olives for decoration

In a deep bowl, combine all of the ingredients except peppers, olives, and parsley, and toss lightly. Cut the red peppers in half with zig-zag cuts. Place the fish mix in each half of a pepper with parsley and olive garnish!

And Gigi said …. *Bon Appétit!*

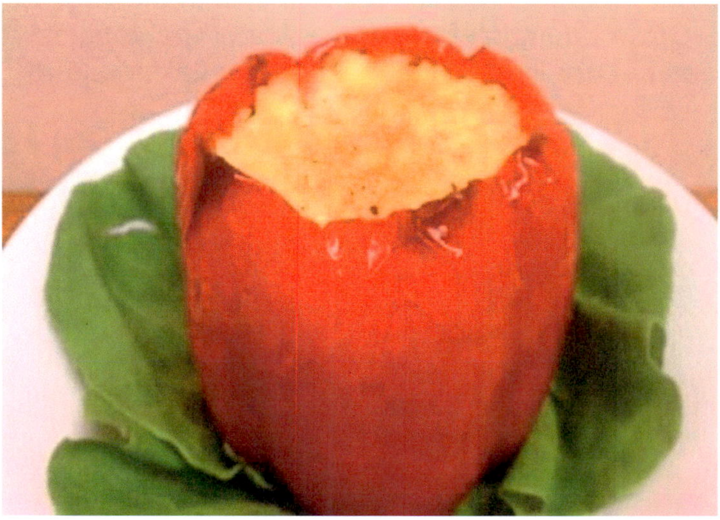

## **Peppers on FISH** (10-minutes from chop to chew)

3-4 fresh fish fillets
1/2 copped red bell pepper
1/2 copped red onion
1/2 copped/sliced cucumber
2 Tbl of wine or orange juice
1/2 lime

Chop up all the vegetables. Pour the wine or OJ in a large skillet pan and turn heat to high. After the liquid boils for one minute, reduce the heat to 75% and lay the fillets down flat and squeeze 1/4 of the lime over the filets /and cover the pan.

Cook for two minutes and then flip over the fillets. Squeeze lime over the fish and cover with the vegetable mix. Cover and cook for 3-4 minutes. (The veggies will get soft but nor limp and the fish will be flaking apart!

Easy Fishy ~ *Bon Appétit!*

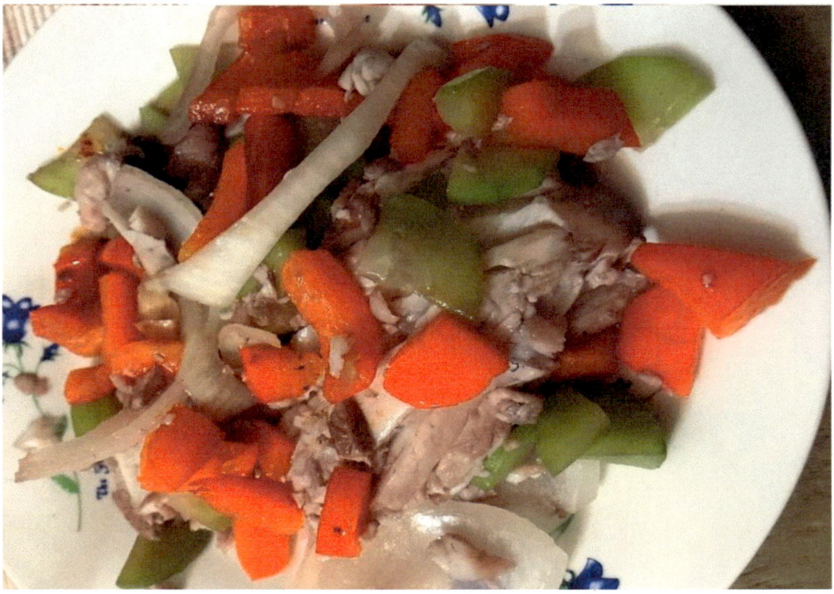

## French Bread with Garlic Crust

Read first before baking to ensure timing.
5-6 c flour
2 packages active, dry yeast
2 c warm water
Sprinkle of cornmeal
1 beaten egg white
1 tbsp water
1 garlic pod, crushed
4 tbsp butter
½ tsp salt

Heat oven to 350º. In large mixing bowl, combine 2 cups flour, yeast, and 1/2 tsp salt, then add warm water. Beat in blender on low for 1 minute and then beat on high for 3 minutes. Work in as much of the remaining flour as possible. Place dough on lightly floured surface. Knead dough for 10 minutes following steps – Flatten – Fold – Flatten – Roll up – Flatten – at least 12 times. Form into a large ball, and place in a large glass container to rise for about 30-40 minutes, cover bowl and place in warm area.

Just before the dough has doubled in size, remove from bowl and place on a lightly floured surface to divide into **2** loaves. After separating roll into two thick loafs, (approximately 3 inches in diameter), place on a greased, double layer cookie sheet (the loaves will lengthen while baking.) Then combine egg white and water and brush onto loaves.

Place in the; bake time of 30 – 35 minutes. After 10 minutes, take out the loaves, make the diagonal surface cuts (1/4 inch deep), and baste on the garlic/butter mix. Place back in the oven. After 20 minutes of total cooking time, again take out the loaves and baste with remaining garlic/butter, then return to the oven. The loaves should be done in 30 – 35 minutes, based on the diameter of the loaves.

*Bon Appétit!*

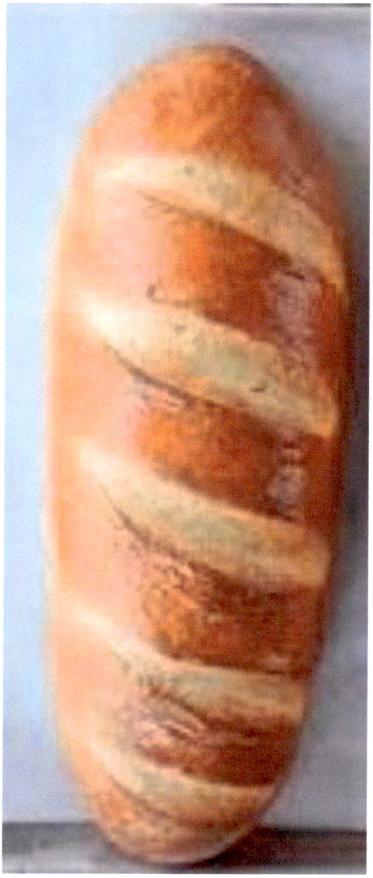

# Gazpacho

1 cucumber, peeled and chopped
6 soft Roma tomatoes, peeled and chopped/blended
2 cloves garlic, minced
1 red bell pepper, seeds removed, chopped
½ red onion, chopped

1½ red wine vinegar
1 tbsp extra virgin olive oil
½ tsp salt
½ tsp black pepper

Separately chop the cucumber, blend the tomatoes, and chop the bell pepper. Mix the dry ingredients, then add the other ingredients and stir vigorously. Refrigerate for 30 minutes (overnight is even better) and serve with gulf shrimp and avocado. Remember one serving is less than 2 cups for victory!

*Bon Appétit!*

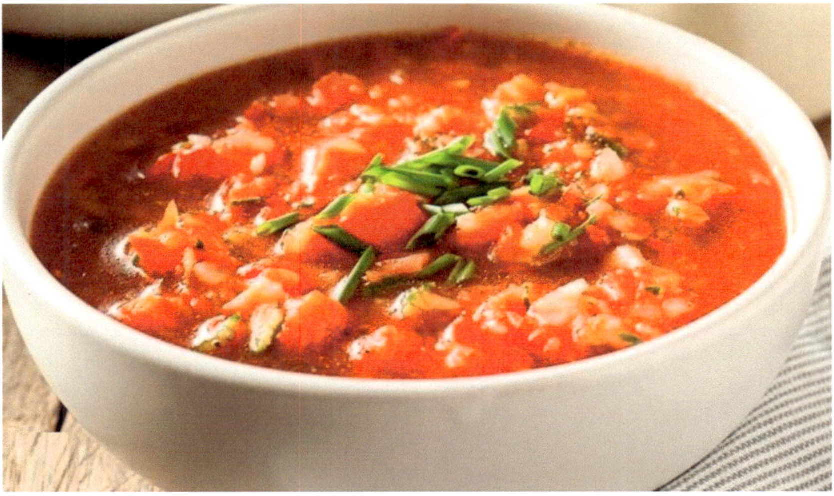

## Gigi's Biscuits (Thanks, Mom!)

Sift together: 2 c organic flour + 4 tsp baking powder + 1 tsp salt

Cut in: 1/3 c organic butter + 2/3 c organic buttermilk

Knead and rollout

Glaze pan with extra virgin olive oil.

Bake at 450º for 8 – 10 minutes (Tasty natural nutrition that her mom baked 100 years ago!) *Bon Appétit!*

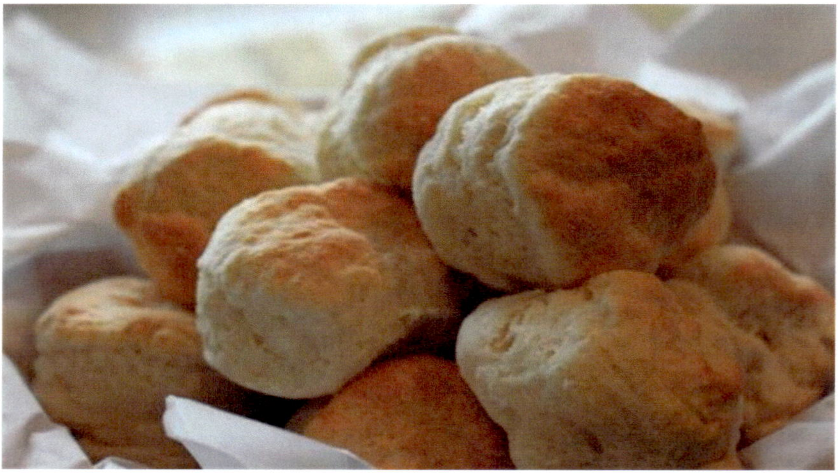

## Gluten Free, Sugar Free Fudge Brownies

Here is a quick recipe for gluten-free, sugar-free, paleo, Rightsize Brownies!

Ingredients

- 1 cup cocoa powder
- 3/4 cup coconut sugar (or Stevia)
- 1 tsp baking soda (1/2 tsp for a more fudgy texture)
- Dash sea salt
- 2 eggs
- 1/4 cup honey
- 1/3 cup coconut oil softened
- 1/2 cup coconut milk
- 1 tsp vanilla extract

Instructions

1. Set oven to 350°. In a mixing bowl or food processor combine all dry ingredients **(cacao powder, coconut sugar/stevia, baking soda, sea salt).**
2. Add the wet ingredients including the eggs, milk, honey, coconut oil and vanilla and blend together.
3. If you are using a keto sweetener or all stevia try adding more milk (1tbsp at each time) to get the idea "fudgy" mixture.
4. Grease an 8x8 Pyrex pan with coconut oil or extra virgin olive oil and pour the batter into the pan.
5. Bake at 350° for about 15-20 minutes until a toothpick inserted comes out dry.

**Serve** with fresh, shredded pineapple, peaches, blueberries, etc.. (Serves 6-8)

Bon Appétit!

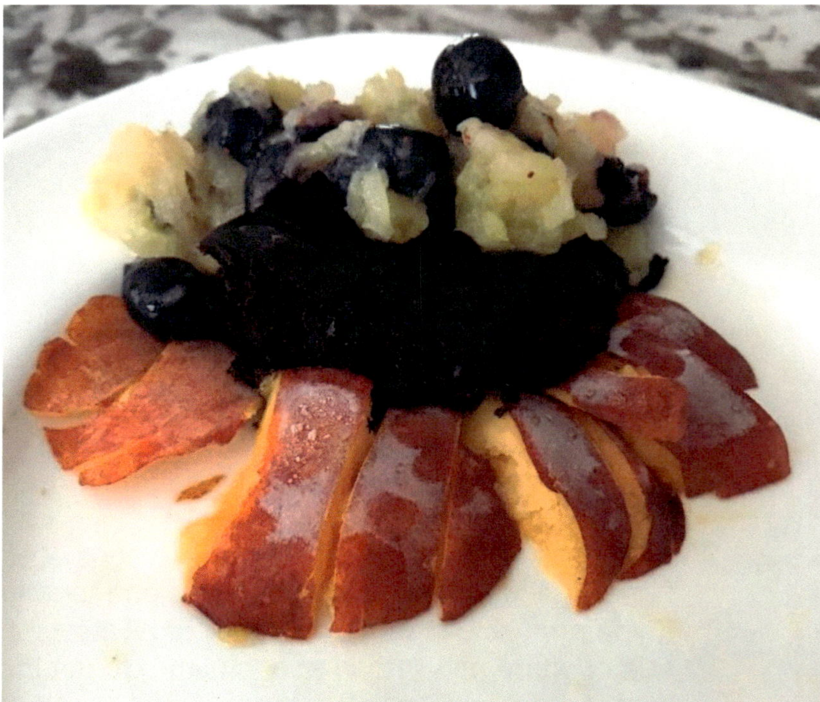

## **Green Eggs & Ham** (Thanks Annie!)

| | |
|---|---|
| Chop | ½ pound of Leeks (1/2 cup) |
| Shred 4oz. Organic Ham | ¼" threads |
| 5 natural eggs | |

Vigorously stir all of the ingredients together for two minutes (see I snuck in an Aerobic-surge!). Then cook as you would cook a large pan of scrambled eggs!

If allergic to Eggs, try 4oz of Eggplant liquefied in a blender.

If allergic to leeks try shredded Kale.

If allergic to Ham, try shreds of Lamb.

*Bon Appétit!*

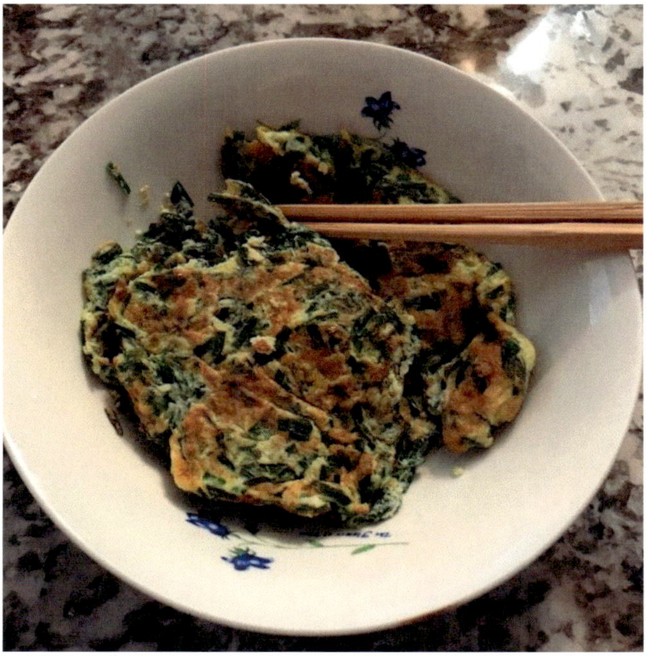

## Ice Cream<u>less</u> Dessert

4-6Peeled, Frozen Bananas

Cacao powder (to taste)

Strawberries (or another tart fruit)

1) Simply peel the bananas in advance (good use of old brown fruit).
2) Place bananas in food processor and blend until smooth.
3) Add cacao (100%) to taste and include or garnish with a tangy fruit like strawberries.

Serve an enjoy or place in a Pyrex pan to serve for later!
*Bon Appétit!*

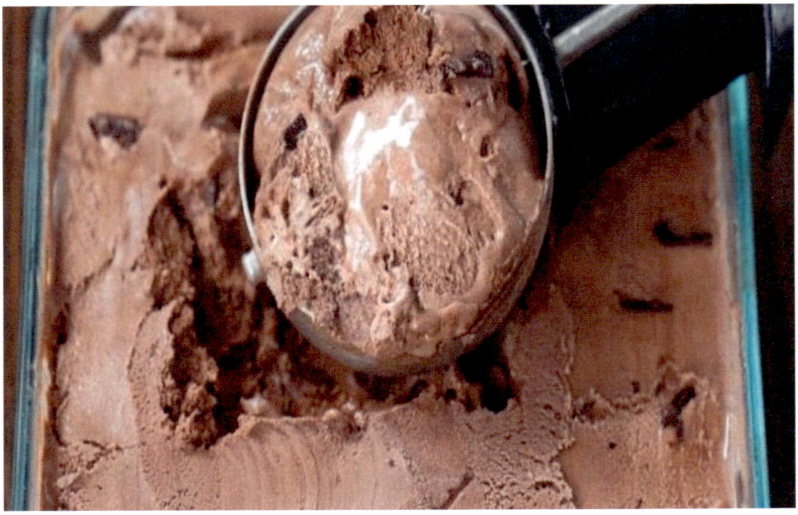

# Island Salsa

Combine the following (use these variables if allergic):

1 diced, large jalapeño, throwing away seeds

½ c chopped kiwi (or mango)

2 c chopped seedless watermelon (or honey dew)

½ finely chopped yellow bell pepper

½ c chopped red onion

1 tbsp fresh chopped cilantro (parsley)

1 sliced and squeezed fresh lime

1 bag organic tortilla strips

*Bon Appétit!*

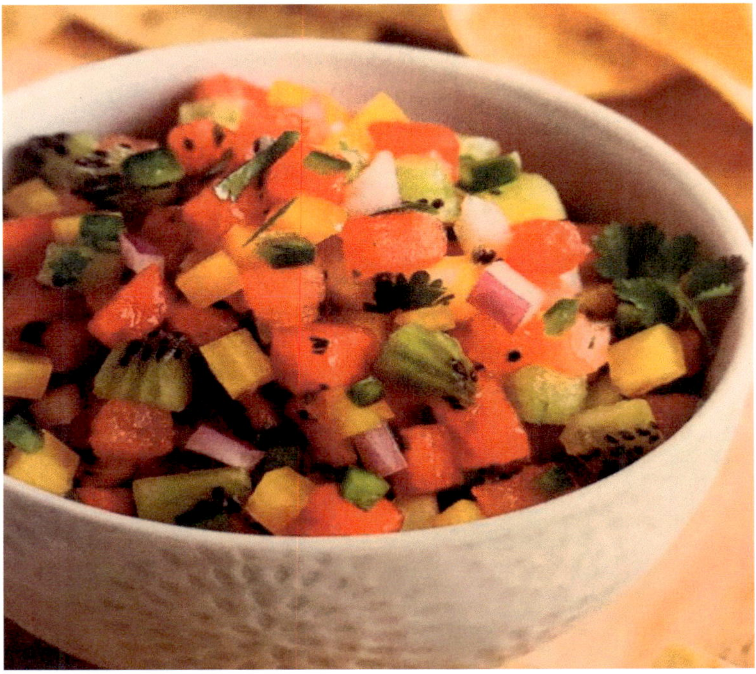

## Kim's Apple Breakfast Quinoa

Need a new breakfast recipe idea? Try Success® tri-color quinoa topped with slow-simmered crisp apples and dried cranberries. Topped with your favorite yogurt.
Ingedients:

1 bag Success® tri-color quinoa
1 cup apple juice
2 tbsp avocado oil
2 tbsp agave nectar
1 large apple, cored and sliced
1/4 c dried cranberries, optional
1/4 c walnuts or almonds
1 c vanilla yogurt, optional

Cooking Directions:

Prepare quinoa according to package directions, adding apple juice to water.
Warm oil and agave in a medium skillet over medium-low heat. Add apple and dried cranberries. Cook, stirring occasionally, until apples are just tender, about 5 minutes. Stir in nuts, if desired. Serve quinoa topped with apple mixture and yogurt, if desired. *Bon Appétit!*

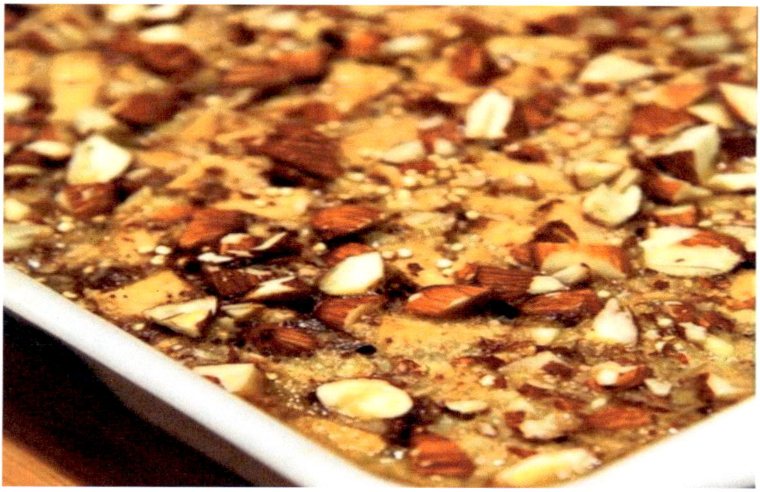

## Kim's Asian Garbanzo Bean Salad

Broccoli. water chestnuts, and garbanzo beans are tossed together with an irresistible sesame-flavored dressing for a quick dish that's delightfully different.

INGREDIENTS

2 cans (16 oz.) garbanzo beans, rinsed and drained
1/2 (6 ounce) box frozen snow peas
1 bag (14 oz) frozen broccoli florets
4 tbsp strong dandelion tea
1 tbsp sesame oil
2 (8 oz.) cans water chestnuts
4 tbsp avocado oil
4 tbsp coconut aminos sauce
4 tbsp sesame seeds
2 tbsp agave
½ chopped cucumber

DIRECTIONS

1. In medium pan, cook broccoli florets and snow peas until thawed.

2. While broccoli and peas are simmering, heat small saucepan over medium heat and add remaining ingredients. Cook until warm. Stirring occasionally.

3. Combine both mixtures, toss and serve.

*Bon Appétit!*

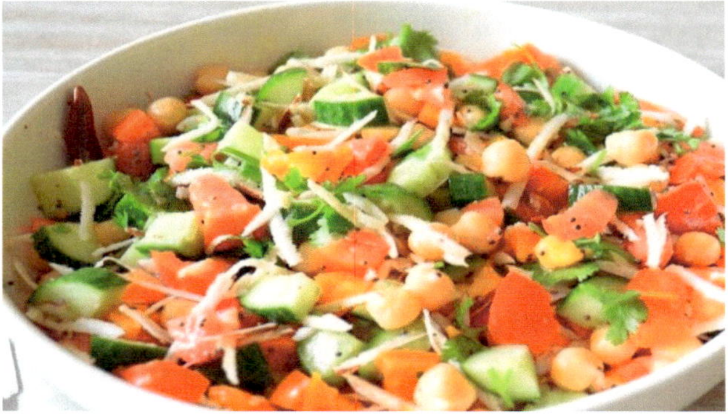

## Korean Pulled Pork

This takes only two minutes of prep time because it utilizes the time-saving power of the crockpot!

- 1 tsp minced garlic
- 1 pork roast
- 1/4 c brown sugar
- 1/2 pear, peeled and shredded
- 2 tbsp Sriracha sauce
- 1 tbsp grated ginger
- 2/3 c organic Korean BBQ sauce (or 1/3 cup Korean teriyaki and 1/3 cup ketchup)
- 1 large carrot, cut into long strips with vegetable peeler
- 1/2 red onion, thinly sliced
- 1/2 English cucumber, thinly sliced
- 1 piece fresh ginger, peeled and cut in half
- 2/3 c rice vinegar
- 1/3 c water
- 3 tbsp sugar
- 2 tbsp Sirach sauce
- 1 tsp salt

Place pork roast in 3 to 4-quart slow cooker. Combine pear, brown sugar, Sriracha sauce, and grated ginger; pour over roast. Cover and cook on low 8 to 10 hours (or on high 4 to 5 hours).

To make pickled vegetables, place carrot, onion and cucumber in non-metal bowl. Combine ginger, rice vinegar, water, sugar, Sriracha sauce, salt, and minced garlic in small saucepan; cook and stir over medium-high heat until sugar is dissolved. Pour vinegar mixture over vegetables, pressing down vegetables to make sure they are covered. Cover and refrigerate at least 1 hour before serving, occasionally stirring. Remove ginger before serving. Remove roast from slow cooker; strain juices and add pear mixture to the meat. Use tongs or 2 forks to pull pork. Stir in Korean BBQ sauce. Serve over hot rice with pickled vegetables on the side. *Bon Appétit!*

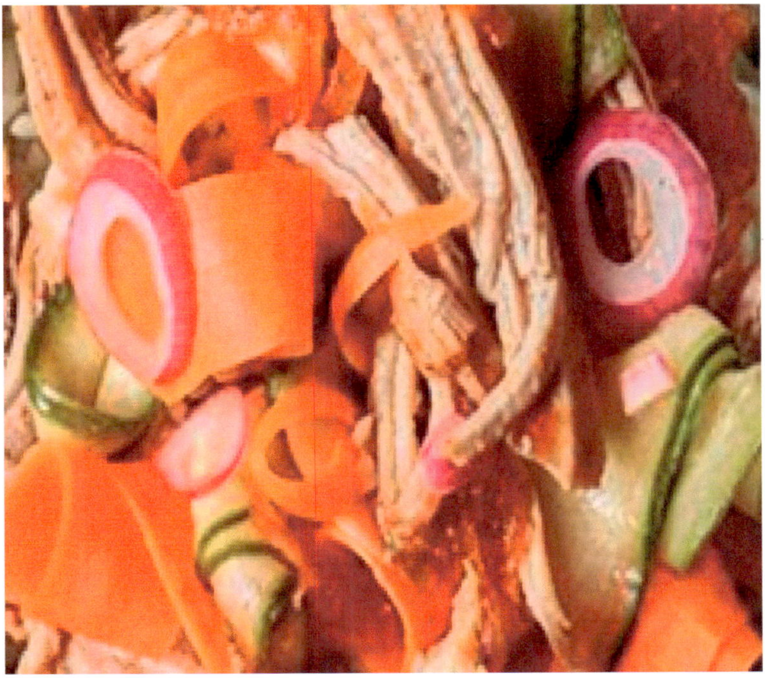

## **Mayonnaise** (Easy!)

(Avoid mayonnaise at restaurants, since most use commercialized, processed mayo for the salad. Even healthy' mayonnaise jars include processed ingredients from high fructose corn syrup to xanthum gum.)

1¼ light olive oil

1 large egg

½ tsp mustard powder

½ tsp salt

Juice of ½ lemon

Place ¼ cup of the oil, plus egg, mustard powder, and salt in a large mixing bowl and mix vigorously for two minutes (energy surge?). While still mixing, slowly drizzle the remaining olive oil into the bowl. After you have blended all of the oil and it has emulsified, add the lemon juice. Blend a few times and *Bon Appétit!*

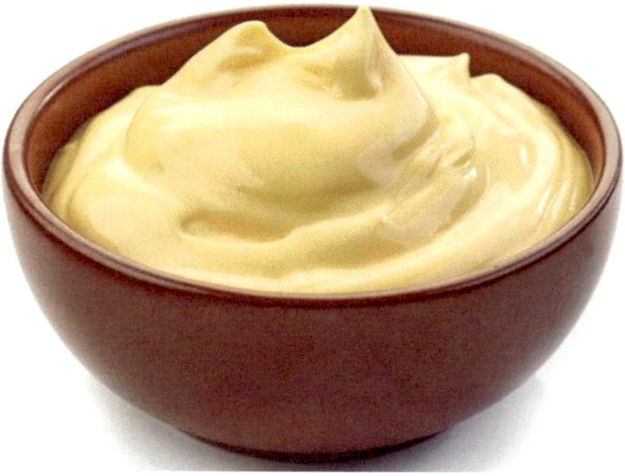

## MEXICAN PORK STEW

This spicy Mexican Pork Stew brimming with pork, sausage, and beans is a classic hearty dish full of deep Mexican flavor and makes for a delicious and easy weeknight meal.

INGREDIENTS

- 1 tbsp. olive oil
- 1 lb. pork shoulder fat trimmed and cut into small cubes
- 8 oz. kielbasa sausage cut into small pieces
- 1 medium onion, chopped
- 3 cloves garlic, minced
- 1 jalapeno pepper, finely chopped
- 1 tbsp smoked paprika
- 1 tbsp chili powder, mild
- 1 tsp ground cumin
- 1/4 tsp Cayenne Pepper
- 1/2 tsp salt or to taste
- 1/2 tsp pepper or to taste
- 28 oz. diced tomatoes (1 can)
- 28 oz. white kidney beans or pinto beans, drained and rinsed (1 can)
- 2 cups beef broth or chicken broth, low sodium
- 4 green onions, chopped
- 1/4 cup fresh cilantro, chopped
- lime wedges for serving

MEXICAN PORK STEW INSTRUCTIONS

1. In a large Dutch oven heavy pot, heat the olive oil over medium-high heat. Add the pork and sausage and brown to render some of the fat from the meat, for about 5 to 7 minutes. Drain the fat, if preferred.
2. Add the onion, garlic, and jalapeno pepper to the pot. Stir in the spices then add the diced tomatoes, beans, and broth. Stir then cover and cook on medium-low for about 25 minutes.
3. Garnish with green onions and cilantro and serve with lime wedges.

*Bon Appétit!*

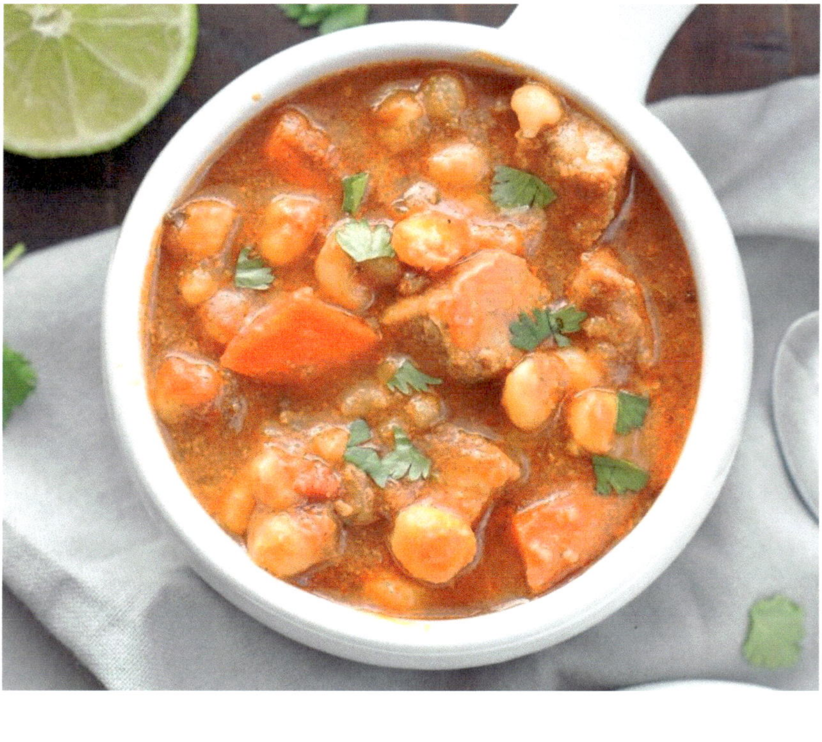

## **No-Mato Sauce** (Kim's Tomato-Free Sauce)

Summary: Use this No-Mato Pasta Sauce in all your recipes that call for tomato sauce. Slather onto pizza dough, spoon onto hot pasta, or dip pita wedges.

Ingredients

- 3 tbsp avocado or sunflower oil
- 1 medium shallot, chopped
- ½ tsp dried thyme
- Pinch of sea salt
- 1 (15 ounce) can pumpkin puree
- 1 can beets (sliced)
- Garnish: fresh chopped basil, parsley and/or oregano, to take it Italian

Instructions

1. Heat olive oil in a large skillet. Sauté shallots and thyme for about 7-10 minutes, until shallots start to brown slightly, stirring often.
2. Add beets to a blender container, put the lid on tightly and whirl until smooth.
3. Add beets and pumpkin puree to the pot, warm and mix with shallots. Add whatever other spices that you need for your sauce. For Italian: add basil, parsley, oregano. For Mexican: add cumin and/or paprika.
4. Sauce is now done, and can simply be reheated for 2-3 minutes, or can be portioned and stored in the refrigerator or freezer for later use.
5. Makes about 4 cups sauce.

The sauce will likely lose its red color the longer you cook it (beets turn brown if you overcook them), so a simple quick re-heat is best. *Bon Appétit!*

# Orange-Ginger Shrimp Skewers

Ingredients:½ c fresh orange juice (2 oranges)
2 tbsp minced green onions
1 tbsp minced, peeled fresh ginger

1 tbsp minced fresh cilantro
2 tbsp rice vinegar

2 tbsp low sodium soy sauce
1 tbsp vegetable oil

2 tsp grated orange rind
1 lb. fresh shrimp, peeled and deveined

4 large oranges, two cut into quarters
1 minced hot red chili (optional)

Directions: Combine all but the shrimp in a bowl and mix. Throw in the shrimp and toss before putting in the refrigerator for 15 minutes to marinate. Remove shrimp from the marinade and alternately place on paired skewers with an orange quarter. Put on a hot grill for 4 minutes on each side and *Bon Appétit!*

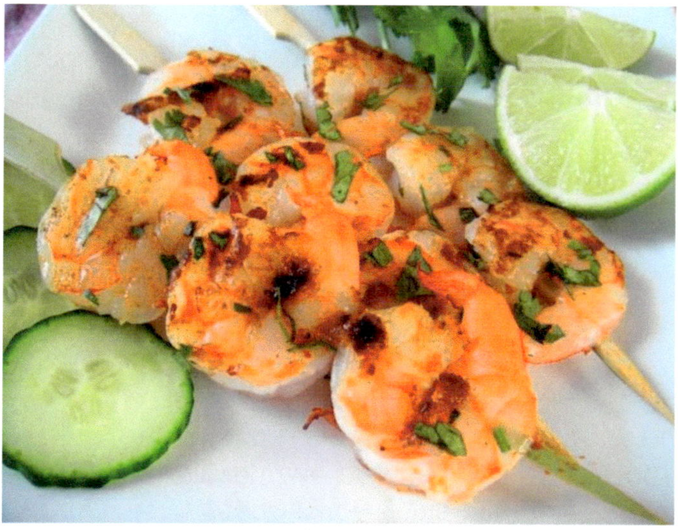

# Poached Fish Filets

4 fresh filets
½ c white wine
¼ c water
8 thin lemon slices, 2 for each filet
1 bay leaf
½ tsp salt
1/8 tsp white pepper
Paprika
1 zested pickle rind
Preheat oven 350º.

Arrange fish in a buttered baking dish.
Combine wine and water and pour over fish.
Arrange filets and cover each with two lemon slices and celery leaves, crumbled bay leaf, salt and pepper. Cover baking dish and poach snapper for 12 min until flaky. Sprinkle with paprika and zested pickle. Eat with roastedvegetables and *Bon Appétit!*

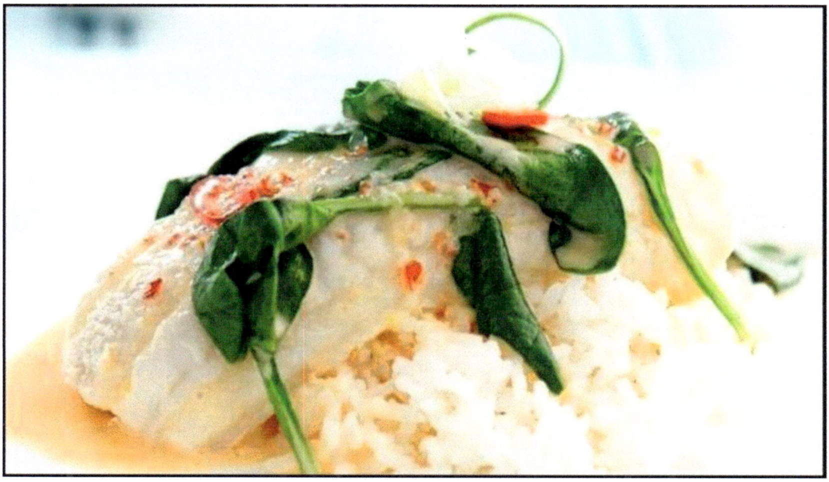

# Quick Salsa

4 ripe (soft) Roma tomatoes
1 c fresh corn
½ red onion, chop before you throw it in the blender
1 jalapeno (I cut in half and remove the core seeds which are the hottest part)
Fresh cilantro

Put in blender and blend with interval speeds (high 2 seconds, off 2 seconds, high 2 seconds, off 2 seconds, etc.) for about 10 repetitions and your salsa is ready!

*Bon Appétit!*

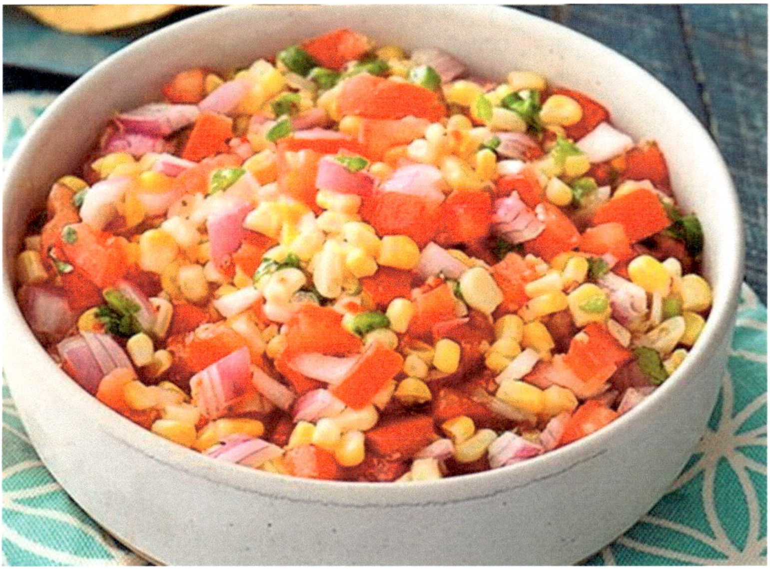

## Salmon Salad

1 ½ lb. fresh salmon fillet, skin on one side

1 c red wine vinaigrette
1 bottle of beer
1/8 c garlic
½ tsp basil
½ tsp lemon peel
½ tsp tarragon
½ tsp black coarse ground pepper
½ tsp cCayenne Pepper
1 tsp orange rind + artsy salad stuff (green leaf lettuce, spinach, red pepper, mini corns, broccoli, red onions, carrot shavings, mini tomatoes, etc.)

1) Mix the dry ingredients to be rubbed on the fish right before you grill. Then soak the salmon in the vinaigrette and beer for *only* 15 minutes before you start to cook it.
2) Make your grill as hot as possible (on our gas grill that equals starting it on high for 5 minutes with the lid closed), so that when you are ready to grill, you cannot hold your hand close to the grill rack for more than a few seconds.

3) Rub the dry ingredients on the meaty side of the fillet, as the other side will go on the grill to be blackened and later removed. Mix the green salad that can be garnished with the crispy, taro shreds.
4) Place the fish on the grill with the skin side touching the grill surface. Close the grill and do not look for eight minutes. After eight minutes have passed, check to see if the fish is flaky. If it is, remove the fish (that will take a strong metal spatula as the skin is blackened onto the grill rack). Then remove the skin, which can be done easily if the fish has cooked enough.
5) Put the fish with the seasoned side up on top of the salad fixings. For dressing, boil the vinaigrette/beer sauce before using it as topping. *Bon Appetite!*

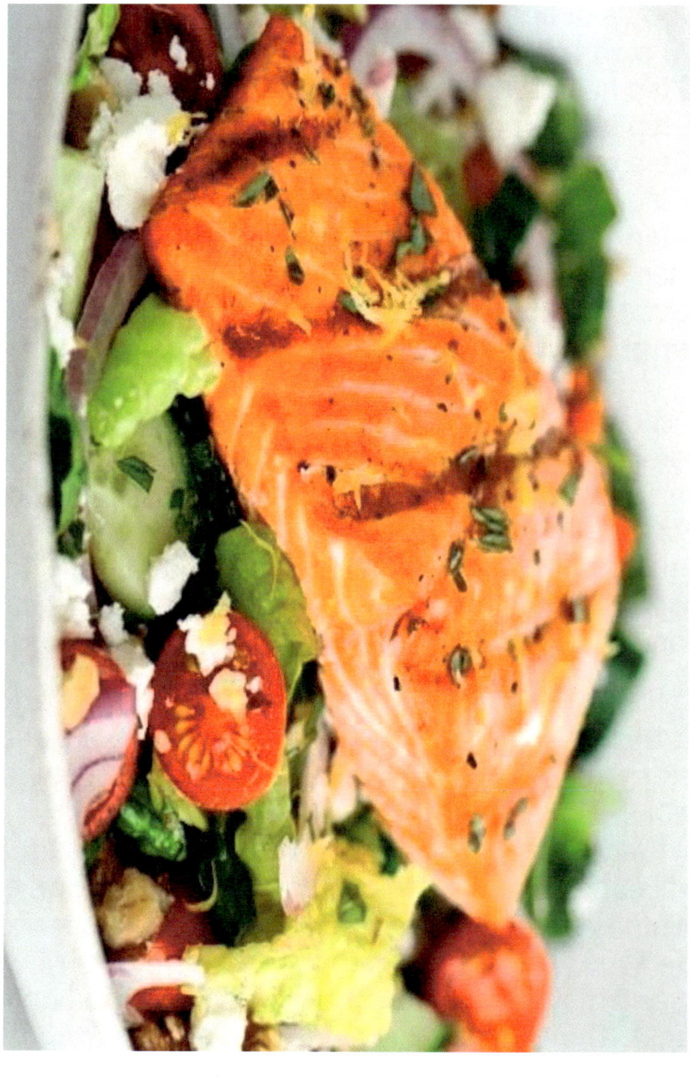

## Shrimp, Leeks, Spinach Pasta

- ¾ lb. gemelli, fusilli, or other (natural) pasta
- 1 lb. peeled and de-veined, fresh medium shrimp (Katie's Seafood, Galveston)
- 2 leeks, white and light green parts only, halved lengthwise then crosswise
- 2 tbsp unsalted butter
- Kosher salt and black pepper
- Finely grated zest of 1 lemon
- ¾ c heavy cream
- 10 oz. baby spinach (12 cups)

1. Cook the pasta according to the package directions; drain and return it to the pot.
2. Meanwhile, heat the butter in a large skillet over medium heat. Add the leeks, ½ teaspoon salt, and ¼ teaspoon pepper and cook, stirring occasionally, until the leeks have softened (3 to 5 minutes).
3. Add the shrimp and lemon zest and cook, tossing frequently, until the shrimp is opaque throughout (4 to 5 minutes more).
4. Add the cream and ½ teaspoon salt to the pasta in the pot and cook over medium heat, stirring, until slightly thickened, 1 to 2 minutes. Add the shrimp mixture and the spinach and toss to combine. *Bon Appétit!*

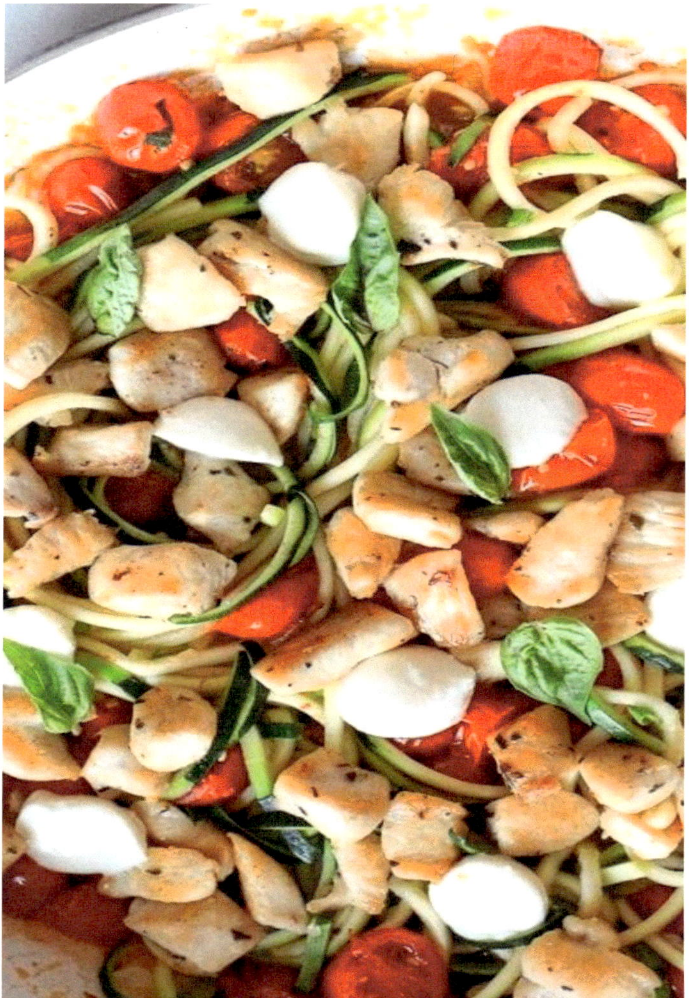

## Southwest Chicken Twist

1) Cook 4 – 6 chicken breasts in the crockpot on high for 4 to 5 hours.
In the crockpot, add 1 cup of orange juice and ½ cup of medium, chunky natural salsa.
2) Combine and cook the following ingredients in a medium covered pot on low for 1 hour:

2 potatoes cut into thin, quarter slices

1 can of black beans that have been washed in strainer

½ of a large red pepper cut into ½ inch strips

2 whole Roma tomatoes with several cuts in the sides
¼ of a red onion cut both into slices and chopped bits
¼ lime squeezed into broth
½ cup of water
¼ cup of watery salsa
1 garlic clove, smashed
1 tbsp spicy organic mustard
3) After the mix has cooked on low for an hour, put in the breasts that you're going to eat at that meal for about 20 minutes, and serve with limes and avocado slices!

*Bon Appétit!*

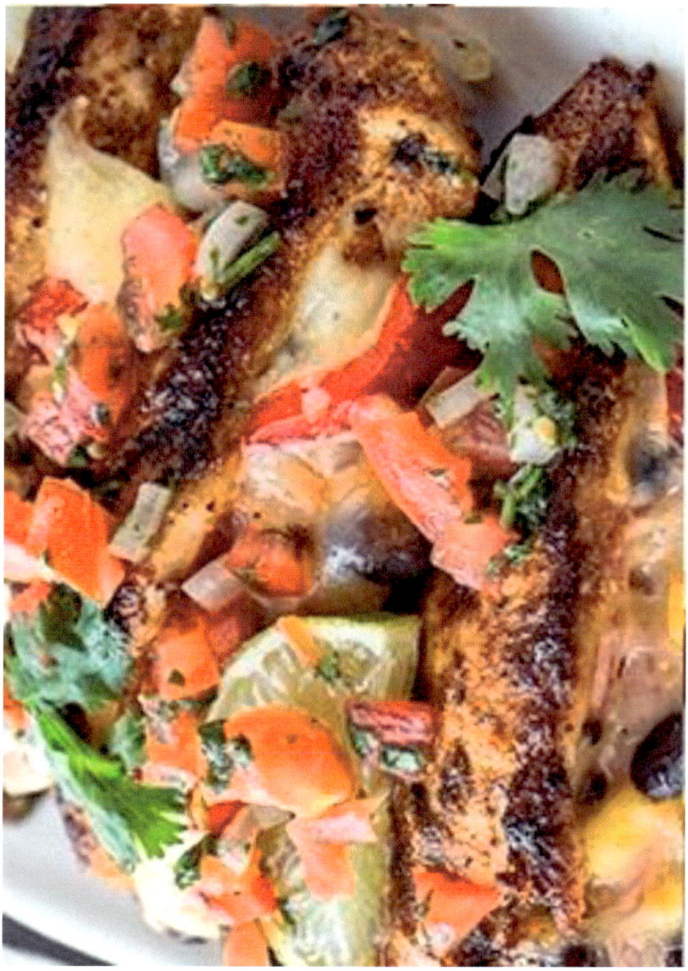

## Spiced Sesame Green Beans

1 lb. haricots verts, trimmed
¼ c organic soy sauce
¼ c rice vinegar
1 heaping tbsp organic almond butter
1 heaping tsp tahini
1 tsp toasted sesame oil
1 tbsp grated fresh ginger
1½ garlic clove, minced
¼ c toasted sesame seeds
1 tsp crushed red pepper flakes
2 tbsp freshly snipped chives.

Bring a large pot of generously salted water to a rapid boil. Add the haricots verts and cook until bright green, about 3 minutes. Transfer to a colander to drain and rinse under cold water.

In a small bowl, whisk together the soy sauce, vinegar, peanut butter, tahini, sesame oil, ginger, and garlic. Pour over the haricots verts and let sit for 20 minutes. Garnish with the sesame seeds, pepper flakes, and chives, and serve. *Bon Appétit!*

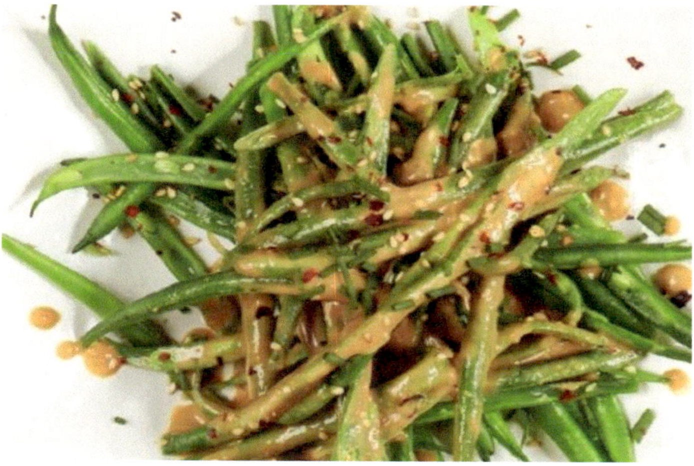

# Strawberry Muffins

3 c all-purpose flour
½ tsp salt
½ c whipping cream
½ stick butter
1 c strawberries
1 c brown sugar
2 tsp cinnamon
2/3 c vanilla yogurt
1 ½ tsp baking powder
2 eggs, beaten
1 ½ tsp baking soda (Extra butter to coat the muffin cups)

Combine dry ingredients in a bowl: Cut in butter with a pastry blender until the mixture resembles coarse meal. Add blueberries and toss. Add yogurt and egg whites, stirring just until the dry ingredients are moistened (dough will be sticky). Coat the muffin tins with butter. This should fill 8 jumbo muffin cups.

Bake at 350° for 25 minutes or until the muffins rise and have a hollow sound when you thump them! *Bon Appétit!*

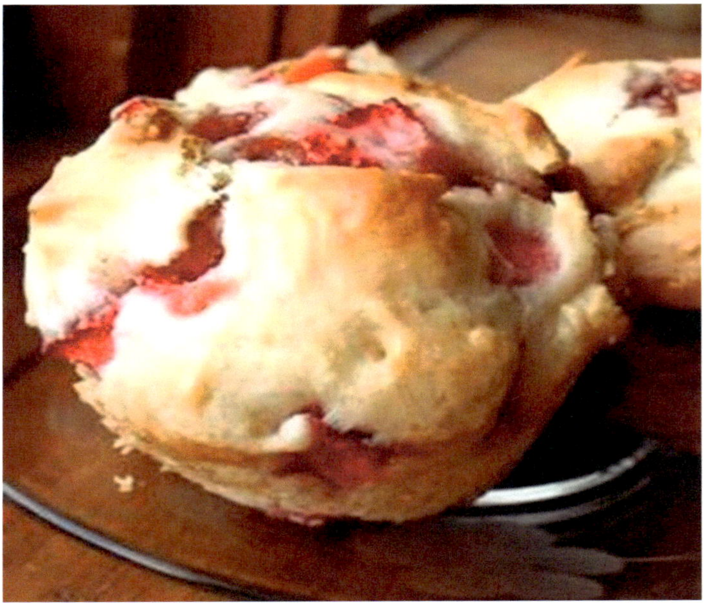

# Island **Steak and Avocados**

2 6-oz tenderloin steaks
1 tsp black ground pepper
2 garlic cloves, peeled
1 tsp salt
2 tbsp extra virgin olive oil
4 tbsp soy sauce
1 avocado, peeled and splint lengthwise
1 shallot, peeled

Remove steaks from fridge for 30 minutes and baste both sides with organic soy sauce. Preheat grill to 500º and oven to 350º. Toss garlic and shallot with 1 tbsp olive oil and place on a roasting pan in the oven for 20 minutes. Then place in a food processor, add the remaining olive oil, and puree. Cook the steaks on hot grill for only 3 minutes/side and then allow to rest unheated for 10 minutes while you roast the avocado. Place the pureed garlic shallots on each steak and enjoy raising your B-12 this weekend! *Bon Appétit!*

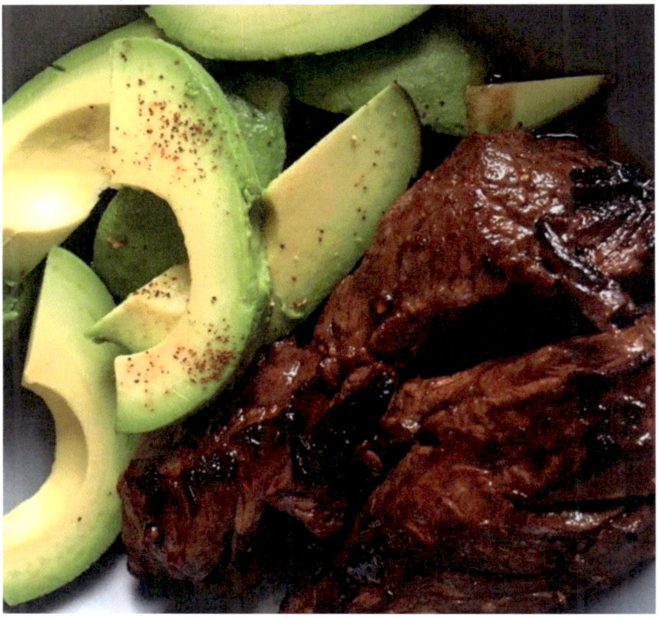

## Taco Cups

This is great for parties or for a quick meal when busy!
(6-cup jumbo muffin tin)
Six 6-inch organic or homemade flour tortillas
Kosher salt and freshly ground black pepper
1 tbsp extra-virgin olive oil
½ onion, finely chopped
1½ tsp chili powder
1 tsp Worcestershire sauce
1½ tsp ground cumin
1 tsp ground coriander
½ tsp dried oregano
½ tsp paprika
¼ tsp garlic powder
12 oz. ground organic beef chuck
1 c black bean and corn salsa
2 c shredded iceberg lettuce
Shredded cheddar
Guacamole
Sour cream, for topping

First lube your muffin tins with butter. Preheat the oven to 425 degrees F. Gently fold the tortillas in half, then in quarters. Place 1 in each cup of the tin and unfold to make a cup. Sprinkle with a pinch of salt. Bake until golden, 8 to 10 minutes. Let cool.
Meanwhile, heat the vegetable oil in a large nonstick skillet over medium-high heat. Add the onion and cook, stirring occasionally, until softened, about 2 minutes. Add the chili powder, cumin, coriander, Worcestershire, oregano, paprika, and garlic powder; cook, stirring, until the onion is coated, about 1 minute.

Remember your pre-grilled beef for the week? Add the beef with salsa and heat. Fill each taco cup with a thin layer of lettuce and then the beef mixture. Top with cheddar, guacamole, and organic sour cream as desired.
*Bon Appétit!*

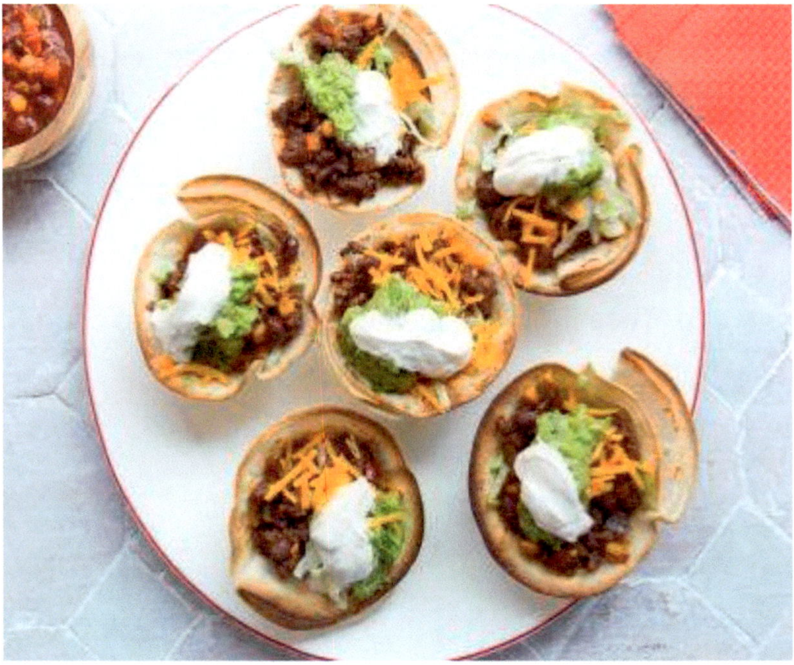

## Zucchini Pasta

5-6 Large Zucchini
3 Tsp Extra Virgin Olive Oil
1 Cup Fresh Basil (or orregano if allergic to basil)
Avocado (if you like)
2-3 Garlic Cloves (Smashed)
1/3 cup pine nuts
1-2 Tsp Lime Juice (better than lemon)

1) Spiral slice the zucchini in the food processor and set aside on paper towels to absorb the extra moistrure.
2) Combine all other ingerdients in teh food processor abd blend into a cream.
3) Toss the zucchini and sauce (also add cherry tomatoes for color and
   *Bon Appétit!*

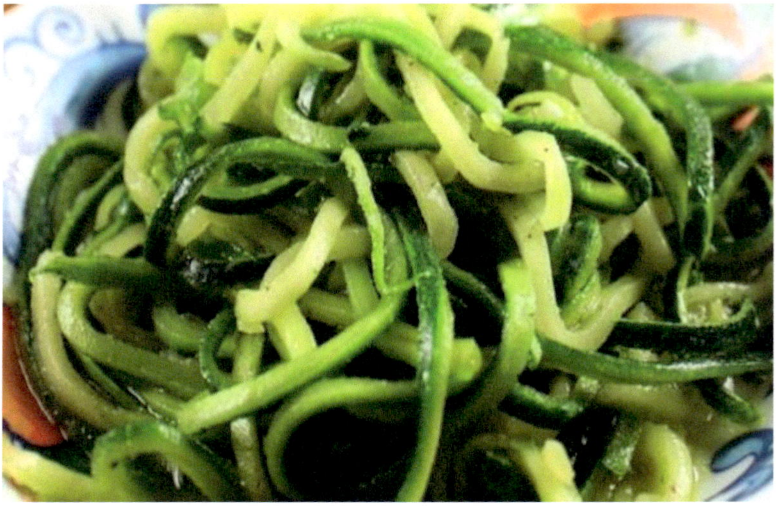

***Digest this***: The right foods can be delicious and you don't need to starve for weight loss. Fasting actually slows the metabolism but eating more often (natural foods) raises the metabolism in multiple ways!

If you have allergies to one food or spice, still make these recipes your own and send to me for our next Recipe book!

# CHAPTER 10

# Nutritional Assessment and Food Allergen Testing

**Taste of Victory:** Here is a dear nurse's victory in losing fat while on 12-hour shifts! "Tina" is a dedicated RN and a mother of four children, and she could never previously reach and maintain her optimal weight loss goal. She worked 12-hour shifts, so she didn't have time for diets or exercise. After testing for food allergies, she eliminated 47 foods, and was also prescribed a lectin-free diet. She simply started taking nuts and other quick snacks to work and ate every three hours unless she was with a patient.

She even dashed to patient calls or did jumping jacks at the nurse's station! The quick two-minute Aerobic-surge exercises, combined with eating quality, clean, non-allergen foods five times a day, worked! In four months, she dropped *4* dress sizes, -26% of her fat mass, -27 inches, and 20 pounds of pure fat!

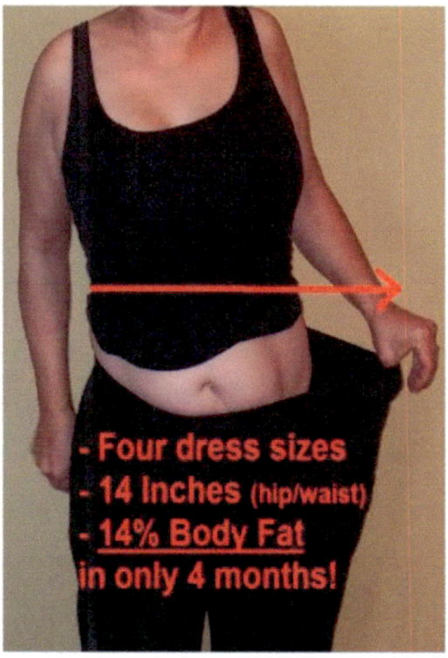


**Your Victory Starts Today!** Start by writing down all of the food that you consume this week, and include snacks as well. Then look back to see how often you are eating, and what quality versus processed foods you have consumed. How many meals left you full and stuffed? How many meals made you feel energized?

How much variety are you seeing in your weekly eating? There are an estimated 250 primary foods (that we will test for allergens). How many of these do you eat regularly? Now ~~cross off~~ those foods that were processed, packaged, or made commercially. These need to be eliminated ASAP. The remaining foods were the only foods helping your metabolic rate, but if you ate more than 2 cups, then even those good foods were pooled with a feeding method that lowered your metabolism.

For Example:

MONDAY

Meal 1 ______________________________

Meal/snack 2 ______________________________

Meal/snack 3 ______________________________

Other foods eaten ______________________________

| **High Glycemic Index Carbs** | | **Low GI Carbohydrates** | |
|---|---|---|---|
| Beer | 100 | Brown rice | 50 |
| HiFructCornSyrup | 100 | Whole wheat bread | 50 |
| Baked Potatoes | 95 | Brand bread | 50 |
| French fries | 95 | Sweet potatoes | 50 |
| Potatoe chips | 90 | Peas | 40 |
| Cornflakes | 85 | Strawberries | 40 |
| Popcorn | 85 | Figs | 35 |
| Sugar | 75 | Carrots | 30 |
| Cola | 70 | Dairy Products | 30 |
| Cookies | 70 | Green beans | 30 |
| Raisins | 65 | Chickpeas | 30 |
| Bananas | 60 | Grapefruit | 25 |
| Long Grain Rice | 60 | **Dark Chocolate** | 22 |
| White Spaghetti | 55 | Tomatoes | 15 |

## Dietary Assessment

Mark each of these foods that you consume D for daily, W for weekly, or leave blank if you eat it less often than once a week.

Apricots
Artichokes
Asparagus
Avocado
Bacon
Bananas
Bee pollen
Brewer's yeast
Broccoli
Brussels sprouts
Buckwheat
Carob
Cod fish
Corn
Cottage cheese
Eggs
Garlic
Kale
Legumes
Lentils
Millet
Mustard greens
Oatmeal
Okra
Parsley
Peanut butter and peanuts
Peas
Pork
Rye
Sunflower seeds
Sesame seeds
Tempeh
Wheat germ

If you are not eating 21 of these each week, then you would probably benefit from taking **L-Carnitine,** which will help boost the metabolism as well.

## The next foods to be analyzed contain Chromium Picolinate.

Banana
Barley
Broccoli
Garlic
Liver
Brown rice
Basil
Green Beans
Mushrooms

Oats
Romaine Lettuce

If you are not eating these foods several times a week, you may have a deficiency in Chromium Picolinate. If so, you might benefit from a scientifically-proven natural supplement, **Metabolic Acceleration**. Also, green tea extract has been shown beneficial in research and one could never drink enough tea to equal the dosage of 315 mg/day.

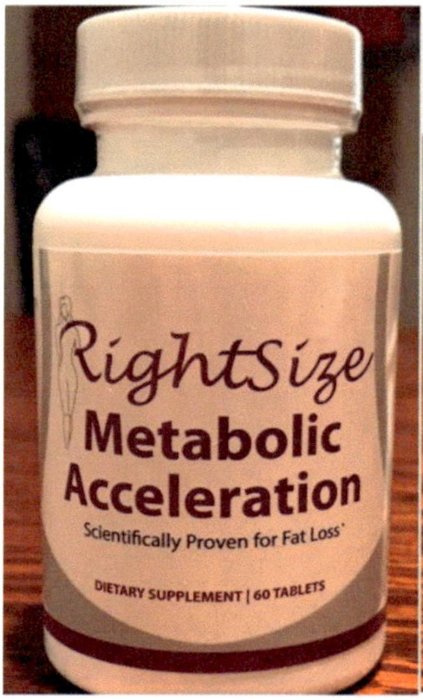


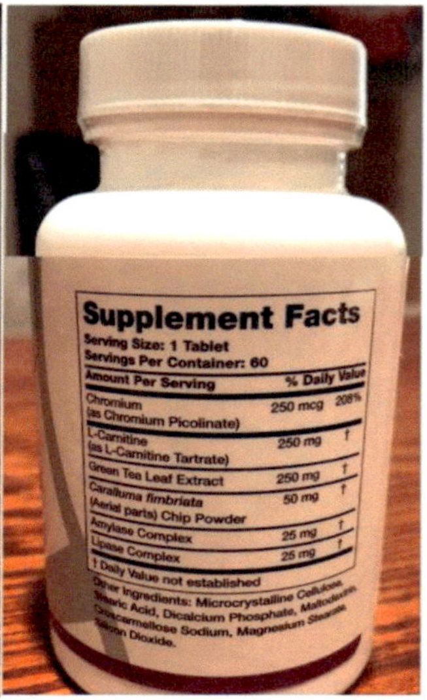

## Enzyme Deficiencies

These deficiencies are common in different ethnic groups of African or Asian descent. Take this quiz to see if this needs to be treated to increase your enzyme production.

1) Please describe your body and when weight is gained.

A. Weight gained evenly (or primarily in stomach area)
L. Carry weight in hips and thighs
P. Carry weight in upper body (stomach up)
C. Remained similar distribution since a teenager, but increased

2) Please circle problems/symptoms you currently experience:

A. Allergies, cold hands/feet, fatigue, headaches, hemorrhoids, low blood pressure, neck and shoulder aches, upset stomach (ulcers)

L. Arthritis, aching feet, bladder iinfections, breast lumps, hay fever, gall stones, hives, jaundice, prostate problems, urinary problems

P. Alcoholism, arteriosclerosis, back problems, constipation, ear infections, heart disease, high blood pressure, insomnia, sciatica, osteoporosis

C. Aching knees, chronic allergies, colitis, Crohn's disease, diarrhea, IBD, milk intolerance

3) Which foods give you problems (such as gas, bloating, nausea)?

A. Carbohydrates (vegetables, breads, pies, sweets)
L. Rich fatty foods or spicy foods
P. Proteins (meats)
C. Dairy

TABLE

A = Amylase Deficiency
L = Lipase Deficiency
P = Protease Deficiency
C = Combination L & P

You can train your body to regain enzyme efficiency and also train your body to overcome low level allergic reactions (after conclusively tested). This is done in a similar manner to how immunologists use weekly allergy shots to desensitize your body's reactions to allergens. Instead of having a "shot of milk" (if you have a low level milk allergy), you should have an exclusive feeding session each day where you consume only 2 tbsp of pure, organic whole milk and 1 tbsp of a non-allergen food, like blueberries. Eat and drink nothing else and this alone will be a controlled meal.

This moves towards the area where you will need a weight loss specialist or nutritionist's instruction but now you get the idea of how we can train your body to become desensitized to certain foods and also increase activity of enzymes like lactase.

## Food Allergen Testing and Elimination

There is more research on using the food allergen identifications for obesity reduction, as it has been used for many years in treating migraine headaches and stomach disorders. You read about our comparison study in 2017 and all of the 17 subjects dropped their weight and fat significantly. The biggest health measure was that their the **BMI values (height/weight) dropped an average of 20%**!

In the following year they averaged financial savings of $1900 each. This is because medication for type 2 diabetes, high blood pressure, cholesterol, chronic pain, etc. were reduced after the overweight disease was cured. Don't we all want to live "Drug Free?"

Lewis, Woolger, and Melillo examined food allergen elimination in another study (2012) for obesity reduction. They tested 120 overweight subjects (mean age 45.5, BMI = 29) for IgG food allergens. Foods that had a positive reaction were removed from experimental subjects' diets for 90 days. These subjects experienced significant changes in weight and waist/hip circumferences. The mean value changes were as follows: weight –5kg, $P<0.01$, and waist circumference -5.4cm, $P<0.01$.

Their IgG test is more specific than the full test of all four reacting immunoglobulins that we use, and their study did not use any other protocols for weight loss as the Willis et al (2017) study did. However, that study shows evidence that proves efficacy of food allergen identification and elimination, in obesity reduction.

You've read that food allergen eliminations help with other conditions too like migraine headaches and irritable bowel syndrome. Why not test to see where you are?

## Why is This Successful?

Let's go back to the beginning description of the immunoglobulin system and reactions (Chapter 5). After successful elimination of the known and hidden causes of this disease, the total number of immune reactions will go down. If we avoid having our regular #1, #2, and #3 reactions, then we will be less likely to have reactions #4, #5, and #6. Does that make sense? The continual reduction in inflammation is also a contributing factor in reducing this disease.

The bottom line is that we want to help you identify the causes of this disease for a lifetime cure!

***Digest this:*** We have to know and counteract the causes before we can be cured!

# CHAPTER 11

## Sexy Foods

**SKIN.** What does your skin need for texture (baby smooth skin), resilience, and reduction of wrinkles? Here are the amino acids (parts of a protein) that your skin needs and then which foods contain

**Argenine** (L-Argenine for humans) helps restore you skin from damage (sunburn, blemishes, dray patches). It is found in these foods:

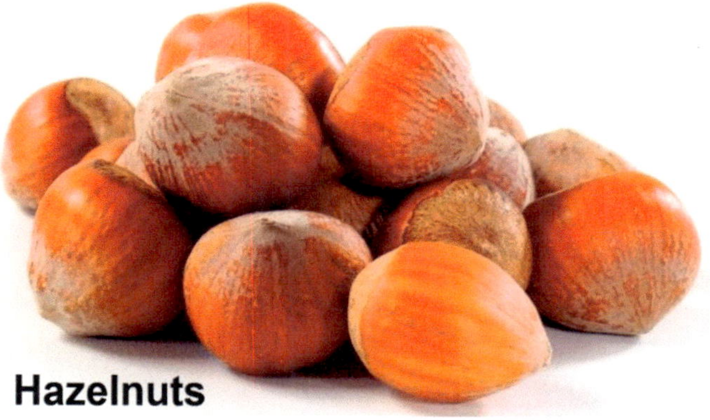

**Hazelnuts**

- Almonds
- Beef
- Brazil nuts
- Brown Rice
- Buckwheat
- Cashews
- Chicken

- Cocoa (only 100% chocolate)
- Dairy Products
- Hazelnuts
- OATS
- Pecans
- Sesame Seeds
- Sunflower seeds
- Walnuts

**Histidine** is a component which works both as an antioxidant and it helps smooth your skin. It is found in these foods:

- Beef
- Chicken
- FishNuts
- Sesame Seeds
- Sunflower seeds
- Whole Grains
- Venison

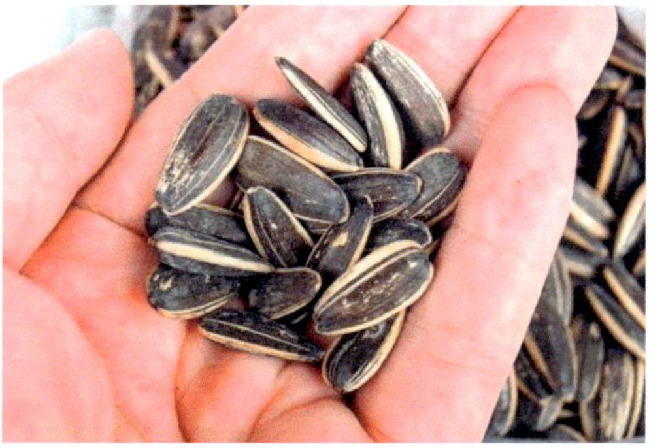

**Methionine** is a structure that protects the skin from harmful substances like chemical or excess sun and it is found in these foods:

- Brazil nuts
- Chicken **Eggs**
- Fish
- Fruits
- Grains (cereal)

**Lysine** strengthens the skin surface by helping build collagen matrix in the skin. (This is also beneficial for healing of cold soars.) This come the following foods: Avocado

- Chicken
- Cottage cheese
- Fish
- Pork
- Red meat

**Proline, leucine and glycine** help reduce the depth of wrinkles and comes from these food sources:

- Dairy Products
- Eggs
- Lamb
- Veal
- Venison

## What about SEX?

**Woman's sexual pleasure** comes first and sexual pleasure for both men and women are linked to good blood flow and connective tissue health. A woman's pleasure is more complex than a man's but studies have shown that treatment with a combination of **L-Arginine, ginseng, ginkgo, damiana,** and other vitamins were beneficial. In a double-blind, placebo-controlled study, 108 women and they measured levels of sexual arousal. Dr. Ito et al examined both pre and postmenopausal women, ages 22-73.

They used surveys to measure 1) "Sexual desire," 2) "Overall Sexual Pleasure," and 3) Frequency of Intercourse as the variables in this study. After four weeks the women treated with the L-Arginine formula showed a 72% rise in sexual desire and overall sexual pleasure rose by 68%. The control subjects who received only a placebo pill had lower changes in sexual desire and overall sexual pleasure but had a greater change in frequency of intercourse.

This study did not control for partner's desire and other There are more variables than just amino acids can improve but every beneficial ingredient will add to the full pleasure for a woman.

**L-Arginine for men** is an amino acid which helps achieve erections. Specifically L-Arginie is the precursor for nitrous oxide (NO) which dilates blood vessels and increases blood flow to fill an erection. Several studies (even studies on "old rat erections") has proposed that the lack of L-Arginine and NO are primary causes of Erectile Dysfunction (ED).

Stanislavov and Rohdewald performed a randomized, controlled double-blind study on 50 men with ED. They treated these subjects with a mixture of Pycnogenol®, roburins, L-arginine, L-citrulline or a placebo for the control subjects. Treatment over one month returned erectile function to normal without side effects.

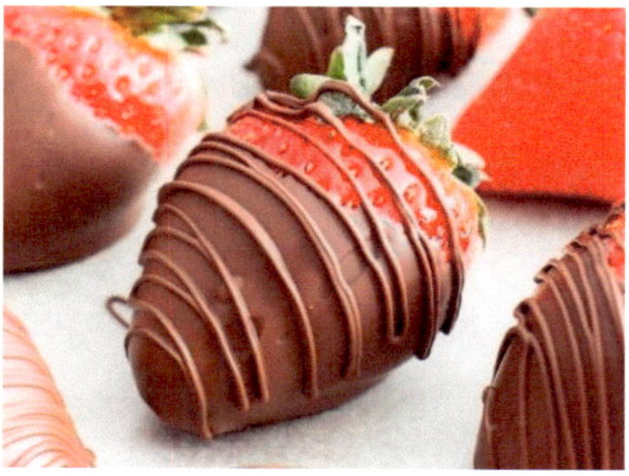

***Diget This*: Sexy Food? Strawberry + 100% Chocolate makes Fat DROP!**

## CHAPTER 12

## How it feels like to lose 4,600 pounds.

**That is how much pure Fat was dropped by my last 100 patients!** Some of these Rightsize Champions were categorically obese and some just wanted to lose a few inches in their waist. (The average is -6 inches.) They all had one thing in common; they did not have success from diets or even hours in the gym. Some had tried pharmaceutical options like Phentermine but that did not work or even more fat came back after the treatment stopped. (It's speed which reduces the appetite and long term results show decreases in bone mass density.)

One champion just wanted to regain her health and the weight loss was just a nice "side effect!" Another is an ICU nurse who didn't have time to go to the gym or eat diet food. She said "I can't describe what it feels like to lose so much fat and it was easy, too easy! But you do have to continue to eat the non-allergen foods and perform the 2-minute exercises for permanence."

What if you wanted to regain the size you wore when you were an AFROTC Cadet? The PAN-5 system was very effective for several of my classmates but permanence only came after they tested to isolate the specific causes of the overweight disease. How can you lose weight if you are having daily inflammatory reactions from hidden food allergens or several reactions each day? One patient had such a problem.

After realizing that she was having reactions to food like broccoli and 40 other common food allergens, she not only lost 60.lbs but had to have her Mess Dress uniform taken in ... four sizes smaller than when she was a young lieutenant!

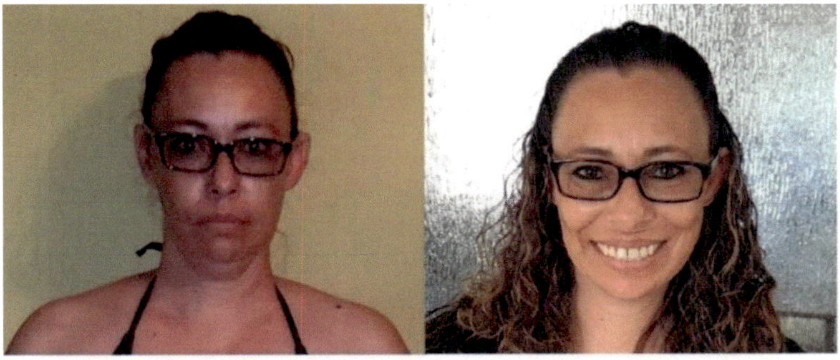

**Dropped 18% of her Body Fat! (never to be found again!)**
**- 4 Dress Sizes, -14 inches (hips-waist-thighs) in FOUR Months!**

Another patient Amy had saved up for a gastric bypass because she had a BMI = 40. After the surgery she had dropped 80.lbs but she complained of the side effects that should could only eat small meals or the pain would make her vomit. She also learned that she could not eat foods with long chain fats like hamburger. She said it seemed worth it until over the next ten years she regained over 80.lbs!

We met an immediately performed the food allergen blood test which showed she had significant reaction to 45 of 250 foods including the “healthy foods” of catfish, garlic, and lettuce. It was a shocker to Amy but she diligently eliminated all of the allergen foods and the weight began to fall of conservatively at -10.lbs/month. As the weight loss slowed she increased the number of her Aerobic-surges from 2-3/day to 5-6 and the weight continued to be reduced.

After nine months she had lost more than she regained and now 12 months later, she is even smaller!

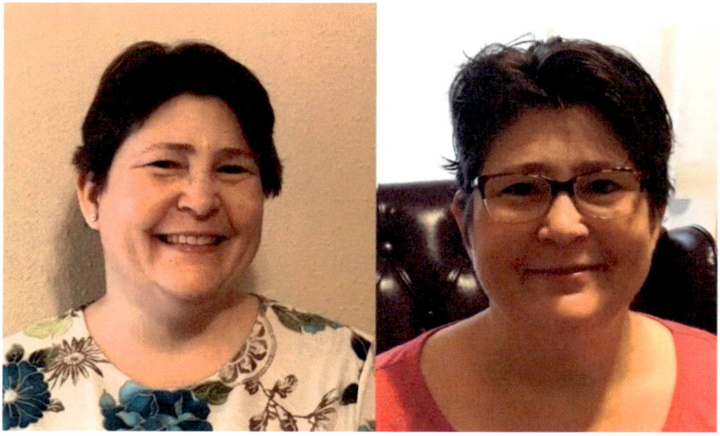

## Great Change!

Jill started with one of the worst looking nutritional assessment surveys but finished with the best example of Eating more often and Exercising Less but more efficiently!

DAY 1

0700 – Chex cereal, coffee extra powdered cream (sodium sulfate cereal, sucralose creamer)
1000 – skip meal (drops metabolism)
1200 - two fast food hamburgers and diet Pepsi (commercial buns, fillers in beef and high fructose corn syrup in ketchup, 4-mel coloring in Pepsi)
1500 – skip meal
1800 – chips, queso, guacamole and four margaritas (Velveeta synthetic products, alcohol slows metabolism and high fructose corn syrup.)

DAY 2

0700 – Coffee double creamer and skip meal
1000 – hard candy (high fructose corn syrup)
1300 – double servings in buffet (TBHQ, meat fillers, HFCS in ranch dressing, etc.)
1600 – Exercise Gym weights for 60 minutes
2000 – Six "light beers" and Mac & Cheese (sulfur dioxide beer and tartazine in mac)

DAY 3

0600 – Coffee double creamer, Packaged muffin on airplane flight (Potassium bromide and TBHQ)
0900 – Taco Bell at arriving airport (do we need to imagine these evil ingredients?)
1200 - Lunch where he spoke and did not eat much
1300 – Hamburger, fries fast food
1800 – three beers, mixed nuts and chips on the return flight (sulfur dioxide beer)

DAY 4

0700 – Coffee double creamer and grabbed an apple on the way out (hooray!)

1000 – Coffee double creamer and skipped meal

1200 – grabbed a pop-tart for road trip (high fructose corn syrup and TBHQ)

1500 – skipped meal

1900 – Pizza homemade (seven hours since last feeding dropped metabolism)

2400 – bacon, eggs, and tequila shots

**AFTER meeting with me** we eliminated foods with over 20 problem foods and drinks with substitutions like Tevia soda instead of Diet Pepsi, organic vs processed ketchup, milk instead of processed creamer, etc. Then we performed a food allergen test of leukocyte reactions (white blood cells) to 250 foods and here are the results.

**Food Allergen Testing (250): Dr FB Willis, Rightsize Clinic 11 May 2019**

| ACUTE | MODERATE | LIGHT |
|---|---|---|
| Agave | Apple | Allspice |
| Avacado | Crab | Ancho Chili pepper |
| Cashew | Cucumber | Arrow root |
| Kidney Bean | Halibut | Basil |
| Sweet Potato | Honey | Black beans |
| | Leaf Lettuce (red/grn | Cabbage |
| | Molasses | Cayene pepper |
| | Pork | Cinnamon |
| | Redbeat | Cumin |
| | Sesame | Curry |
| | Spelt | Hops |
| | Yeast | Jalapeno |
| | Yellow Squash | Lamb |
| | | Oyster |
| | | Peanuts |
| | | Rye |
| | | Sorghum |
| | | Vanilla |
| | | White Potato |
| N = 5 | N = 13 | N = 19 |

While having 37 food allergies might seem scary, it is good news because now we know the causes of the overweight disease for Jill beyond the poor food choices.

**Her new start** began by eliminating the acute and moderate allergens for the first two weeks, and then we eliminated all 37 for her lifetime plan. The foods underlines in Red were actually foods that he ate in the 4-day food tracking. Let's look left to right and discuss how we exchanged the food allergens with the healthy foods which we call "Green foods."

Since avocado was in the guacamole at the bar, I suggested he stick to one bowl of chips and home-made salsa which is even tastier. Instead of the small package of “mixed nuts he ate when flying, I suggested he make a snack pack of almonds, walnuts, and pine seeds. The lettuce on his burger needs to be eliminated but I suggested having more red onions and tomatoes.

**Without yeast** Jill still could enjoy bagels, homemade tortillas, crackers, etc. I told her we don’t need to be “Carbophobic” but we do need to make sure she is no longer eating the processed foods (packaged muffins) or hamburger buns. She loved eating one, full **burger taco** with beef, lots of veggies and salsa on top instead of ketchup.

**Alcohol** - I told Jill it would be the best start to eliminate all alcohol for the first month and this was a challenge. However, she got used to drinking a glass of carbonated water with limes and then later would just drink one glass of red wine. (This eliminated the hops.) Allspice is a potential problem because while we can avoid a certain food when we are dinning out, the spices are hard to detect until it’s too late. For all of the spices, I gave Jill a card which listed all of the Spice Allergies and she gave that to the chef whenever she went to a restaurant.

Obviously fast food chains have all of the food prepared in plants away from the restaurant but this was also a good excuse to dine at more of the quaint, charming Mom n Pop restaurants. **When she cruised to Cozumel, she continued to lose weight!**

Here is the food/exercise schedule that gave her great victory in dropping weight, 32% Body Fat, and **Cut her Dress Size in Half!**

**NEW DAY 1**

0700 – Scissor Kicks and fresh strawberries. Coffee with cream
1000 – Water bottle "Floor to Ceiling" lifts and then 1.5 cups Almonds, blueberries
1300 – Climbed 90 steps up the stairs and ate 2 cups of fish, salsa, chips, veggies
1500 – Jumping jacks in the bathroom and ate one peach with a few walnuts with green tea
1800 – Aerobic Threshold bicycle riding at gym before going out with friends to eat Mexican food at a small cafe. Chicken fajitas, corn tortillas, salsa, red onions, with one glass of red wine

**NEW DAY 2**

0700 – Squiggle Jumps before eating 2 scrambled eggs and onions
1000 – Scissor kicks at her desk before eating mango slices that she baked
1200 – 120 Arm Curls (in the parking lot before meeting with the president of her company) then she ate sushi after she gave her Spice Allergen card to the chef
1500 – 120 Stairs and ate  cup of red grapes
1800 – After getting home she Ball Pushups before eating a delicious meal of fresh veggies and grilled fish

**NEW DAY 3**

0600 – Heel Raises before even getting out of bed! Then she ate fruit and organic cereal.

0900 – Clock Swings (she has two 5.lb dumbbells that live in her trunk now!) She ate two handfuls of nuts and fruit.

1200 - She did 120 Scissor Kicks as soon as she got to the airport. (An older lady told her she was proud of Jill!) She ate one chicken fajita taco before getting on the plane and enjoyed her stash of LARA Bars when traveling.

1600 – Side Plank for 2 minutes at the hotel and then she ate fish tacos with colleagues.

1900 – Squat Pops before she went and joined her colleagues for one glass of wine with mushroom crepes!

**NEW DAY 4**

0700 – 100 Milk Shakes Coffee with milk and "berries cereal" with pistachio nuts.

1000 – 90 Shoulder Extensions after she parked and then two LARA bars.

1300 – 100 Jumping jacks in the bathroom of a restaurant and her colleague joined her! (Now they have the eternal joke of "bathroom jumping time!" Then she ate fresh snapper and sautéed asparagus.

1600 – Scissor kicks and she ate a pear before going home.

1900 – Jill's niece was spending Friday night and they both had tons of laughs while they did Roll ups together! They baked their own organic pizza!

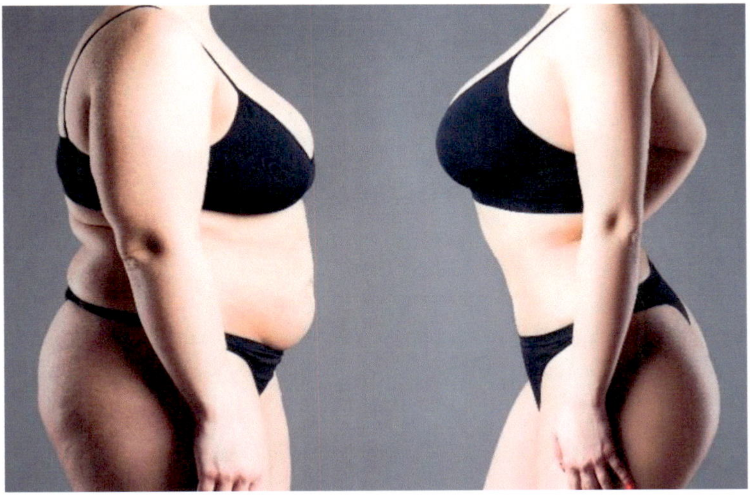

Yes you can really eat pizza to lose weight IF you're not allergic to allspice, garlic, yeast, peppers, tomatoes, etc.

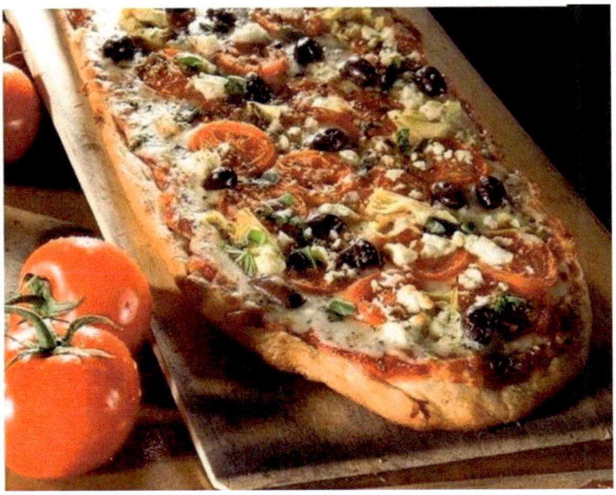

## More Victories!

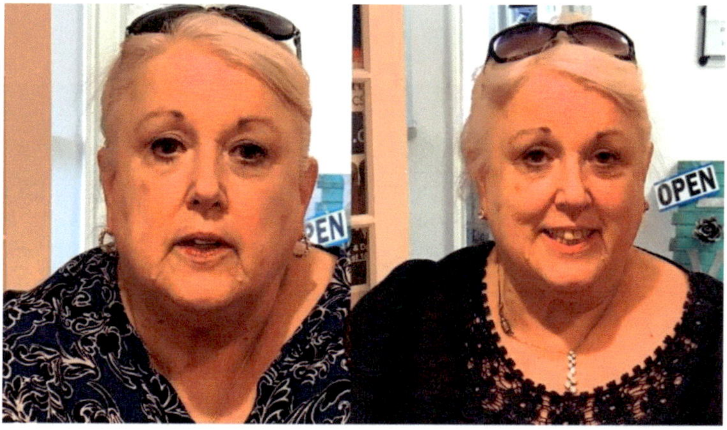


-20lbs, -26 Inches, -8% Body Fat in 60 Days!

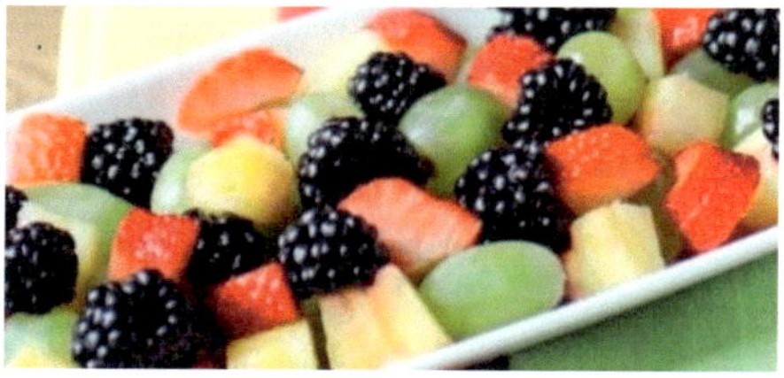

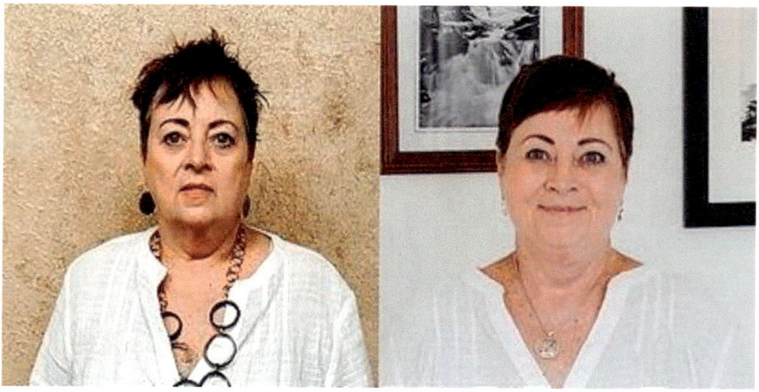

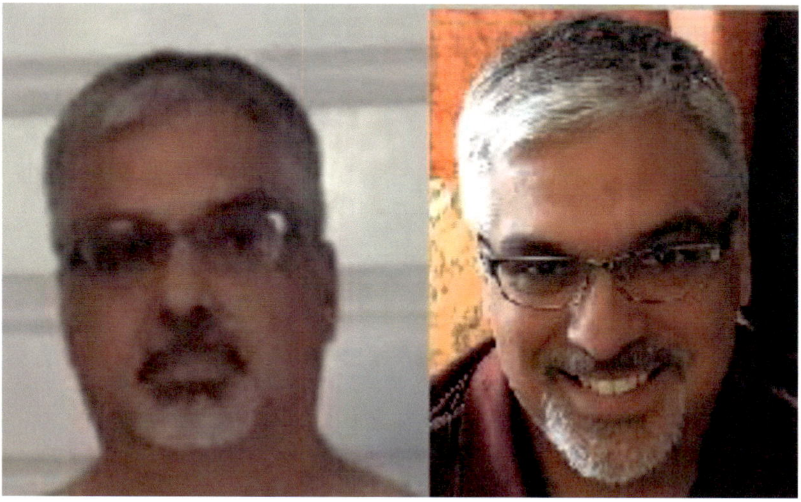

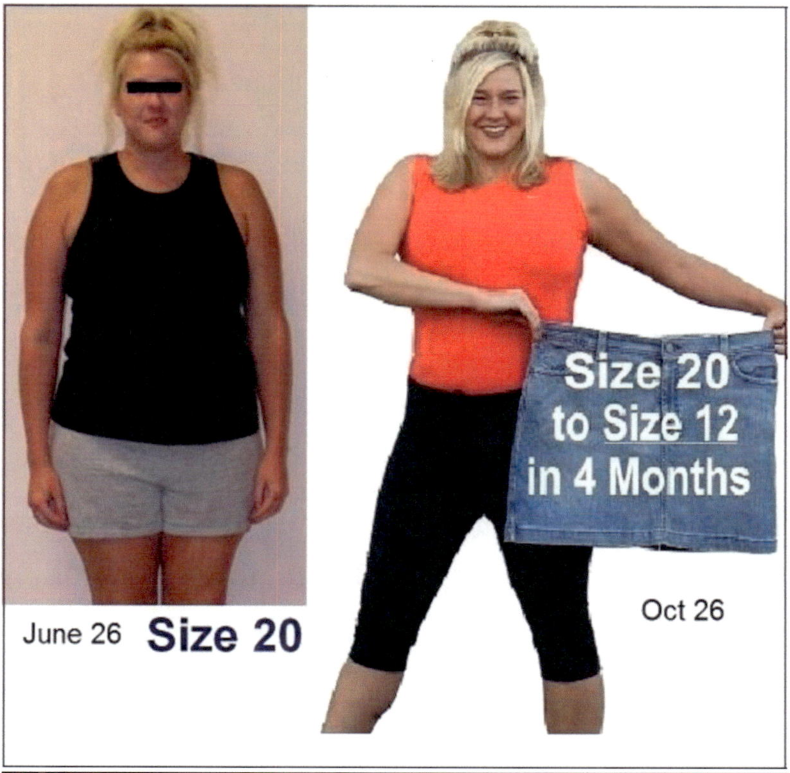
Size 20
to Size 12
in 4 Months
June 26
Size 20
Oct 26

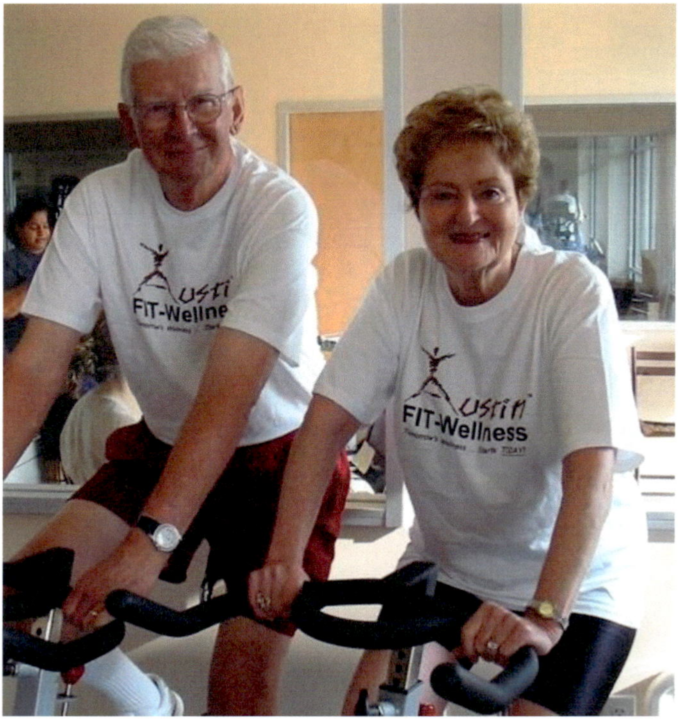


What will be your long term effects of eating clean food with smart exercise? These were Doc's parents who served as a Civil Engineer and a Foodservice teacher! They loved living life with lots of travel and friends, plus they and described themselves as "International Foodies!"

Mom had Alzheimer's but she passed in a way that was perfect for her. She was surrounded by family and she even sung a hymn in her last month, and all of her clothes were "too big". They were the definitive loving parents!

***Digest this***: Each victory preceeds the next!

# CHAPTER 13
## The 30-Day Cure

**Taste of Victory at Any Age!** "Lorraine" had tried a dozen "diets" over the last 50 years until she found that "food was the answer" to both the cause of her overweight disease and her cure! She had tried numerous diets before but they always failed because the cause of her overweight disease was never identified or eliminated. When she started at 75 years of age, over half of her body weight was made up of fat (51.5%). Testing for hidden food allergies and enzyme deficiencies showed reactions from the "healthy foods" (spinach, trout, black tea) she ate regularly. Fifty-six hidden food allergies (of 250 tested) were identified as the cause.

In two months, she dropped -22% body fat and lowered her blood pressure by 20%. After six months, she showed a 40% change in fat mass and she was taken off medication for high blood pressure and type II diabetes. **She went from size 16 to size 6 for her 76$^{th}$ birthday!**

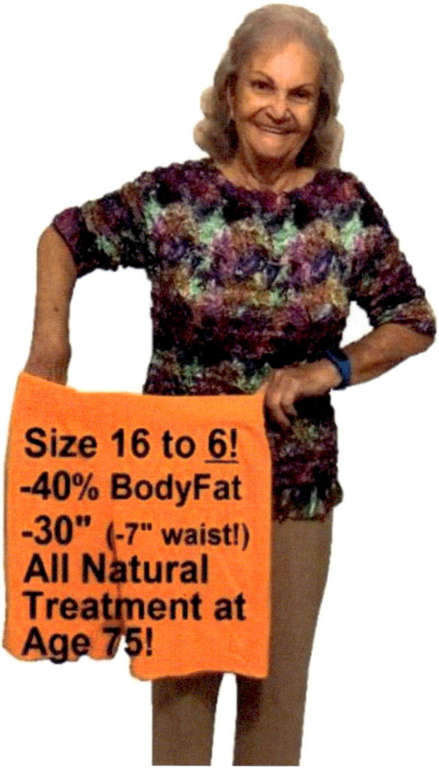


**Start by measuring your Body-Summation (last page) so you will have more variables than just 'the scale' (weight) to measure your fat loss**. Actually fat is the lightest substance in your body, so testing one's body composition is important. A Bod Pod can be used and is located in most major cities: https://www.cosmed.com/en/contact-us/test-site-locator If that is not accessible, you can also get accurate readings of change from a bioelectrical impedance machine.

Bioelectrical impedance (BIA) uses a low-voltage electrical signal to measure differences in bone plus lean body mass vs fat. It requires electrodes at both the feet and hands. (Scales that say they reads 'body composition' are ridiculous.) Omron.com has good equipment that shows valid change however, the pure accuracy will be off by 4-5%. https://omronhealthcare.com/?s=body+composition

Both BodPod and Omron BIA are far better than the old caliper method. I would only count the caliper method accurate if you're an athletic trainer who tests 100 obese patients every day. Test first thing in the morning before any exercise or eating, and then put your scale in the garage for a month.

Start every day in the pages below by planning and "forecasting" your day with
5/5/5 (five aerobic surges and five single Portion meals meals/snacks which include five natural foods) and then at night check off what you actually completed. Achieving 5/5/5 will bring about significant change. Call us at 1-409-632-7131 to get your blood test to accentuate your change and/or make it permanent!

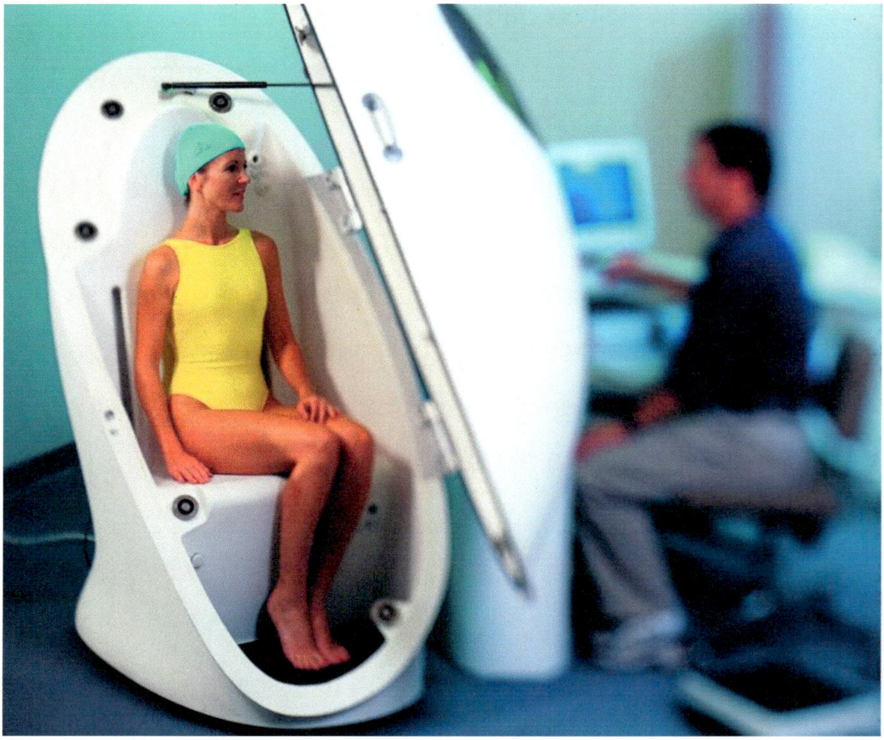

BodPod Body Composition chamber

**DAY 01**

Each day will include "Tips for Success." Use five different aerobic surges (if possible) and eat a different main meal every day. (Make sure you never eat the same food twice a day or two days in a row, to avoid developing sensitivity to any food.

**Tips**: Consult your primary care physician before starting any weight loss program. Today clean your colon of the chemicals and preservatives which have been shown to leave residual traces in the lower GI. Drink 8 ounces of magnesium citrate (laxative), plus 8-12 ounces of water at bedtime to clean out all of the residue from your colon. (Do this on Friday night at bedtime because you will be 'handcuffed to the commode' for a few hours the next morning.) Remember that natural foods can accelerate fat loss! Earth foods are our friends. So on your first day, chose only raw, earth foods for three of your five meals or snacks today.

**DAY 1 Aerobic-Surges:**

1) (Scissor Kicks)
2) ______
3) ______
4) ______
5) ______

**Meals and Snacks:**

1. ______
2. ______
3. (Caribb Wings)
4. ______
5. ______

Each of us will have challenges on this pathway, so write them down here and then later write how you turned that challenge into a resounding Victory!

**Challenges:**

**Victories:**

**Day 02**

**Tips**: Have you ever felt bloated or gassy after eating a specific food? If you have one symptomatic food allergy, then I bet you have another 20 hidden food allergens. Hellen Keller once said, "The most beautiful things in the world cannot be seen or touched, they must be felt with your heart!" Listen to your body more closely.

**Aerobic-Surges:**

1) (Bicycle Sprint) __________

2) __________

3) __________

4) __________

5) __________

**Meals and Snacks:**

1. (Doc's Energy Bars) __________
2. __________
3. __________
4. __________
5. __________

**Challenges:**

**Victories:**

**Day 03**

**Tips:** Make time to just “be”! Take a quiet walk at sunrise and enjoy the day! Even if you are in the mountains or downtown, go to a quiet, natural area or garden and just breathe in the beauty our world gives us! Then plan your success and get success from your plan!

**Aerobic-Surges:**

1) (Arm Pedal) ____________________

2) ____________________

3) ____________________

4) ____________________

5) ____________________

**Meals and Snacks:**

1. ____________________
2. ____________________
3. ____________________
4. ____________________
5. (Annie’s Sautéed Pork) ____________________

**Challenges:**

**Victories:**

## Day 05

**Tips:** Have a joyous day and make that choice! Remember the *intensity* of your energy surge should equal to quickly finishing the fifth flight of stairs. Your heart rate is elevated (if you're not on beta blocker medicine like propanolol) and your breathing is faster (short of breath), but you're not sweaty. Can you do 120 Glute Bridges fast enough to get you to this level of energy used?

**Aerobic-Surges:**

1) ____________________

2) ____________________

3) ____________________

4) ____________________

5) (Ball Push Ups) ____________________

**Meals and Snacks:**

1. ____________________
2. ____________________
3. (Beach Bean Peppers) ____________________
4. ____________________
5. ____________________

**Challenges:**

**Victories:**

## Day 06

**Tips:** Cherish what you have and where you are today instead of concentrating on what you don't have! At least we can face these challenges, because there are no challenges when you're "six feet under"! Steve Jobs once said, "Your work is going to fill a large part of your life, and the only way to be truly satisfied is to do what you believe is great work. And the only way to do great work is to love what you do. If you haven't found it yet, keep looking. Don't settle. As with all matters of the heart, you'll know when you find it." Work on victory and love each step ... even the stumbles!

**Aerobic-Surges:**

1) (Back Row) ________________

2) ________________________

3) ________________________

4) ________________________

5) ________________________

**Meals and Snacks:**

1. (Blueberry Sweet Bread) __________
2. ________________________
3. ________________________
4. ________________________
5. ________________________

**Challenges:**

**Victories:**

## DAY 07

**Tips:** Know that you *will* have stumbling blocks! It's when you will have challenges, and not 'if.' So you have to plan that into your program. What will you do if something pushes you off your RightSize formula? The first thing you should do is *call us* at (409) 632-7131. Let's work through this together. If you slip and accidentally eat a food that you're allergic to and gain weight, then we'll discuss how to overcome that setback with body works and eating more of your non-allergic foods (six per day)!

**Aerobic-Surges:**

1) (Bed Drapes) ____________________

2) ____________________

3) ____________________

4) ____________________

5) ____________________

**Meals and Snacks:**

1. ____________________
2. ____________________
3. (Caribb Wings) ____________________
4. ____________________
5. ____________________

**Challenges:**

**Victories:**

**Day 08**

**Tips: Turn Up the Heat**! Eat one tablespoon of chopped green or red chili peppers on your food to raise your metabolism (if allergic, choose another pepper). Again this is taking your body to the 'fight or flight' response. Let's not just exist in this life, but live it 110% to the fullest! Colossians 3:23 says, "Whatever you do, work heartily, as for the Lord and not for men."

**Aerobic-Surges:**

1) ______________________________

2) ______________________________

3) ______________________________

4) (Biceps Curls with Water Bottles) ______

5) ______________________________

**Meals and Snacks:**

1. ______________________________

2. ______________________________

3. (Chalupa Compuesta) ______________

4. ______________________________

5. ______________________________

**Challenges:**

**Victories:**

## Day 09

**Tips:** Remember that every time you accomplish one of the PAN-5 variables, you will experience metabolic acceleration! Including one of the foods to accelerate fat loss will help even more. When you forecast your meals for today, add apples, asparagus, and carrots to different meals.

**Aerobic- Surges:** Schedule one before each meal, using energy surges similar to this example:

- AM: Scissor Kicks (ensure aerobic threshold)
- Mid-Morning: 50 Dumbbell (DB) curls alternated with 50 Brain Busters
- Lunch: 100 Steps Upstairs (downstairs doesn't count)
- Afternoon: Shoulder DB Lifts. Perform as many as you can, then rest 5 seconds and continue the next set lifting in front of your body for as many as you can. Then alternate back to lateral lifts until you reach 90 reps.
- Evening: Bicycle sprint for 2 minutes and then cruise back home.

**DAY 09 Aerobic-Surges:**

1) ________________________________

2) ________________________________

3) (Brain Busters in bathroom)

4) ________________________________

5) ________________________________

**Meals and Snacks:**

1. ________________________________
2. ________________________________
3. (Chicken Chili)
4. ________________________________
5. ________________________________

**Challenges:**

**Victories:**

**Day 10**

**Tips:** Chose to see victory! What you expect is what you will receive. Shake off negativity. If you say to yourself, "Oh no, I will never lose this weight and I may gain some…" then *that* is what you will receive. Prophesize, predict, and proclaim your victory by today repeatedly saying, "I may have had problems in the past but I *claim* my Rightsize victory … today!" Five times today say, "I claim victory!"

**Aerobic-Surges:**

1) ______________________________

2) ______________________________

3) ______________________________

4) ______________________________

5) (Clock Swings)________________

**Meals and Snacks:**

1. ______________________________
2. ______________________________
3. (Chicken Tee Pee)______________
4. ______________________________
5. ______________________________

**Challenges:**

**Victories:**

## Day 11

**Tips:** Don't forget that ladies have and need optimal testosterone levels too (ask for labs close to you).

Henry Ford once rightly said, "Whether you think you can (do it), or you think you can't ... you're right."

**Aerobic-Surges:**

1) ______________________________

2) Forward Lunge down the hall) ______________________________

3) ______________________________

4) ______________________________

5) ______________________________

**Meals and Snacks:**

1. ______________________________

2. ______________________________

3. ______________________________

4. (fresh fruit and nuts, try macadamia nuts,mangos!)

5. ______________________________

**Challenges:**

**Victories:**

## Day 12

**Tips:** How can we help our neighbors? Tell them of your immediate success and invite them to share this victory with you! What is the last time you hosted an "all natural" cook out?

**Recipes:** Let's talk about the difference between lean and fat fish. What is the difference? Fish with a higher fat content (good fat) are darker and with a stronger flavor, such as bluefish, herring, mackerel, salmon, sturgeon, and whitefish. These are the best fish to grill or broil because they remain moist. Lean fish like catfish, cod, flounder, haddock, red snapper, sea bass, and perch are better poached, steamed, or baked with basting to keep them from drying out.

**Aerobic-Surges:**

1) ____________________

2) (Incline Chest Press – leaning back at your desk) ____

3) ____________________

4) ____________________

5) ____________________

**Meals and Snacks:**

1. ____________________
2. ____________________
3. (Crockpot Lasagna Soup) ____________
4. ____________________
5. ____________________

**Challenges:**

**Victories:**

**Day 13**

**Tips:** We need to make sure that we have adequate prebiotics in our *RightSize* plan. What are prebiotics? **Prebiotics** are carbohydrates that cannot be digested by the human body, and they are food for probiotics the 'good' GI bacteria. The primary benefit of probiotics and prebiotics appears to be helping you maintain a healthy digestive system.

How can we benefit from probiotics? By increasing the population of 'good' bacteria, it also reduces the bad bacteria in our system for better, more complete digestion. The best source of natural probiotics are yogurt with "live or active culture" or soft cheeses like Gouda. Even sourdough bread from Patty Cakes has probiotics!

Foods rich in prebiotics include asparagus, artichokes, bananas, oatmeal, and legumes. You can purchase prebiotics and probiotics through us or from your local vitamin store.

**Day 13 Aerobic-Surges:**

1) ________________________________________

2) ________________________________________

3) ________________________________________

4) (Jumping Jacks in the bathroom at work!)

5) ________________________________________

**Meals and Snacks:**

1. (Gigi Biscuits)
2. ________________________________________
3. ________________________________________
4. ________________________________________
5. ________________________________________

**Challenges:**

**Victories:**

## Day 14

**Tips:** Today we'll talk about the "**Low glycemic index**," which is the score of a food's ability to immediately raise one's blood sugar. (See page 163.) Remember when we discussed hidden food allergies and I said, "One man's dessert is another man's poison?" For glycemic index, remember, "Not all carbs are equal!"

The GI scale ranges from 1-100, with 100 being an immediate rise like the evil and useless high fructose corn syrup (HFCS)! (Table sugar or ice cream are not this high as they only have a GI score of 75.) The lower GI values are for foods (including sweets) that take a longer time to break down and thus have a slower effect on one's immediate blood glucose levels.

Peaches, strawberries, and mangos have 'low GI' scores of 55 or less. Remember your first morning energy surge, then "one bite" and I suggested strawberry - this is why! Look over the GI scales (chapter 14) and you can see that lots of fruits are actually low GI vs processed breads that are high!

**Day 14  Aerobic-Surges:**

1) (Milk Shakes) ________________

2) ________________

3) ________________

4) ________________

5) ________________

**Meals and Snacks:**

1. ________________
2. ________________
3. ________________
4. ________________
5. (Fish and Sweet Potatoes) ________________

**Challenges:**

**Victories:**

**Day 15**

**Tips:** *When in doubt… move it out!*

That was what I used to preach to my students at McMurry University. Even with my vertebral and shoulder fractures, I still do that. When I went to Walmart to get a toy for my loving Great Dane this weekend, instead of fighting to park close, I parked at the furthest light pole (no problem in forgetting where I parked!). Then I measured how fast I could speed walk back to the door. After 90 paces, I had an elevated heart rate! That didn't count for a 2-minute energy surge, but it helped energize my afternoon! Two laps and it's an energy surge!

**Aerobic-Surges:**

1) ________________________________

2) (Pushups ~ lean against your desk and do 120!)

3) ________________________________

4) ________________________________

5) ________________________________

**Meals and Snacks:**

1. ________________________________

2. ________________________________

3. (Fish Peppers ~ I'm jealous!)

4. ________________________________

5. ________________________________

**Challenges:**

**Victories:**

## Day 16

**Tips:** We need to talk about hidden food allergies again. One patient had her food allergies tested mid-way through her program and found healthy foods like grapes were an acute allergy. So we eliminated all grapes (and wine) and without doing anything differently, five pounds just dropped off in a little more than a week!

**When we eat allergy foods, an inflammatory reaction occurs** and the release of C-reactive protein (CRP) and Immunoglobulin G (IgG) antibodies are tripled, which takes the body from "fight or flight" and pushes the body into "survival, detoxification" mode! This is the "leaky gut syndrome" that you've heard of. Eliminate *all* of your food allergens for victory! First prevent adding weight to lose more weight!

**Day16 Aerobic-Surges:**

1) (Reverse Plank Walk-Around) ________

2) ________

3) ________

4) ________

5) ________

**Meals and Snacks:**

1. ________
2. ________
3. ________
4. (French Bread with Poached Fish) ________
5. ________

**Challenges:**

**Victories:**

## Day 17

**Tips:** Remember that your energy surges four to five times per day are the dependent variable for change! You have to perform these to get the metabolic acceleration for weight loss! Live in the moment and don't worry about tomorrow because tomorrow will have its own challenges. Live today with purpose, joy, love, and with each conscious thought; give it all you have!

**Aerobic-Surges:**

1) ______________________________

2) ______________________________

3) ______________________________

4) (Roll-Ups with the kids!) ______

5) ______________________________

**Meals and Snacks:**

1. ______________________________
2. ______________________________
3. (Island Salsa on anything) _______
4. ______________________________
5. ______________________________

**Challenges:**

**Victories:**

## Day 18

**Tips:** Remember as soon as you awake to immediately do something to accelerate your metabolism! (Try 100 Brain Busters! If you get tired, do 10 jumping jacks before you go back to brain busters.)

Then immediately eat one bite of "fuel" (a few blueberries), particularly if it will be a few minutes until you eat breakfast! **Stay off the scale.** Even if your jeans are tight one day, stay dedicated to the pathway you are on! This is a 90-day journey and you won't reach the goal until then!

**Aerobic-Surges:**

1) ______________________________

2) (Shoulder Extensions right when you get to work)

3) ______________________________

4) ______________________________

5) ______________________________

**Meals and Snacks:**

1. ______________________________

2. ______________________________

3. ______________________________

4. ______________________________

5. (Gazpacho with your sweetie at sunset)

**Challenges:**

**Victories:**

**Day 19**

**Tips:** Try to use different muscle groups for your sequential five energy surges. Instead of climbing 100 Stair Steps, five times a day (downhill does not count), use your core muscles twice, legs twice, and arms once, like this sequence:

- 0700 Scissor Kicks (abs)
- 1000 Stair Climb (legs)
- 1300 Biceps Curl + Triceps Extension in Superset (arms)
- 1600 Indoor Cycle (legs)
- 1900 Toes to the Sky (core)

**Aerobic-Surges:**

1) (Child Curls ~ Aaron laughed buy I got HR up!)
2) __________
3) __________
4) __________
5) __________

**Meals and Snacks:**

1. (Kim's Apple Quinoa)
2. __________
3. __________
4. __________
5. __________

**Challenges:**

**Victories:**

**Day 20**

**Tips: Build yourself up!** Plan your victory and have victory from your plan! Kevyn Aucoin said, "Today I choose life. Every morning when I wake up I can choose joy, happiness, negativity, pain... To feel the freedom that comes from being able to continue to make mistakes and choices - today I choose to feel life, not to deny my humanity but embrace it."

**Aerobic-Surges:**

1) (Side Scissor Kicks) ______

2) ______

3) ______

4) ______

5) ______

**Meals and Snacks:**

1. (Boiled egg) ______
2. ______
3. ______
4. ______
5. ______

**Challenges:** (Love and Hate Scissor Kicks?)

**Victories:**

## Day 21

**Tips:** In October 2016, I intentionally put on 20 pounds by reversing my protocols. (I ate twice/day, non-organic meals, and exercised at the gym 45 minutes each day). Then I reversed and returned to using my PAN-5 and food allergen elimination methods and before Christmas, I had lost 25 pounds and 25% body fat! I watched labels and I did eat delicious sweets (chocolate on coconut; thanks Madison!).

Remember the first month is often for cleansing, detox, and teaching your body to burn fat as fuel. The second and third months are when the most significant change happens, after your body has adapted to the change!

**Tips:** The RightSize method is not hard, but it takes persistence for victory!

Dark chocolate is okay! Read that again, but only if it is 100% cocoa with no sugar or additives. Try eating it with a tart fruit like Strawberry or raw mango!

**Day 21 Aerobic-Surges:**

1) ___

2) ___

3) (Squats)

4) ___

5) ___

**Meals and Snacks:**

1. ___

2. ___

3. (Mexican Pork Stew)

4. ___

5. ___

**Challenges:**

**Victories:**

## Day 22

**Tips:** Remember 5/5/5 and don't short your victory - it's only ten minutes a day!

Try the NEW Bed Drape + Heel Raises! You can perform this in bed laying fully supine (on your back) with just the edge of your butt on the bed. Hold your legs out straight for a minute and then raise both feet together to the ceiling. Do this 60 times and if you can't do the full 120 reps, then hold your legs extended for another 60 seconds!

**Aerobic-Surges:**

1) (Superwoman or Superman; do it together!) ____

2) ____

3) ____

4) ____

5) ____

**Meals and Snacks:**

1. ____
2. ____
3. (Garbanzo Bean Salad) ____
4. ____
5. ____

**Challenges:**

**Victories:**

## Day 23

**Tips:** A victor reminded me that we need to discuss your aerobic threshold (AT) again. The aerobic threshold is when your body consumes the most amount of oxygen and is the only training zone that burns *fat* as the primary fuel. Your AT is 75% of your maximum heart rate (220-age). The envelope for increase or decrease is only 5 beats per minute. If you need to use a heart rate monitor to stay in the zone, Walmart has a heart rate monitor for just $10!

**Aerobic-Surges:**

1) ______________________________

2) ______________________________

3) ______________________________

4) ______________________________

5) (Pop Squats) ______________________________

**Meals and Snacks:**

1. ______________________________
2. ______________________________
3. ______________________________
4. (Korean Pulled Pork) ______________________________
5. ______________________________

**Challenges:**

**Victories:**

## Day 24

**Tips:** A day of rest is good once a week, but if you stop your energy surges, you cannot afford to eat processed foods! I choose 5-5-5 every day and that keeps my step quick and my stomach small. If you take a day off of Aerobic-surges then eat only raw foods with 8 oz. water!

**Aerobic-Surges:**

1) ____________________

2) ____________________

3) ____________________

4) (Squiggle Jumps with kids)

5) ____________________

**Meals and Snacks:**

1. ____________________

2. (No-Tomato Sauce with organic pasta)

3. ____________________

4. ____________________

5. ____________________

**Challenges:**

**Victories:**

## Day 25

**Tips:** We're all conditioned to want a quick change. Previous 'diets' may provide a quick change by shocking the body, but any weight lost is often regained … plus more! Rather than calling this a 'diet,' consider the RightSize to be a marathon race not a sprint. We're teaching our bodies to consume fat as fuel and giving ourselves tools to use down the road, so that when something slows down our metabolism, we'll be able to pick it right back up!

**Aerobic-Surges:**

1) (Toes to the Sky - how many?) ____________
2) ____________
3) ____________
4) ____________
5) ____________

**Meals and Snacks:**

1. ____________
2. ____________
3. (Korean Pulled Pork) ____________
4. ____________
5. ____________

**Challenges:**

**Victories:**

## Day 26

**Tips:** Food allergy testing is needed to help determine the causes of the overweight syndrome or we'll constantly be treating the symptoms instead of the cause! Did you know that several foods, like tomato skins, have lectins which are poisonous to insects? So you may not be "allergic" to such foods, but it takes your metabolism to the floor as your body is only focusing on detoxifying and eliminating the poison!

**Aerobic-Surges:**

1) ______________________________

2) ______________________________

3) ______________________________

4) ______________________________

5) (Toe Taps) ______________________

**Meals and Snacks:**

1. (fresh fruit with boiled eggs) ______________
2. ______________________________
3. ______________________________
4. ______________________________
5. ______________________________

**Challenges:**

**Victories:**

## Day 27

**Tips:** See the sunrise in every challenge! Be still and Listen. Pray and believe that you have received it and the answer shall be yours!

Buddha once said, "(If) Thousands of candles can be lighted from a single candle, and the life of the candle will not be shortened. Happiness never decreases by being shared." Say that again out loud!

**Aerobic-Surges:**

1) ______________________________

2) ______________________________

3) (V-Tucks) ______________________________

4) ______________________________

5) ______________________________

**Meals and Snacks:**

1. ______________________________

2. ______________________________

3. ______________________________

4. (Orange Shrimp Skewers) ______________________________

5. ______________________________

**Challenges:**

**Victories:**

## Day 28

**Tips:** Let's not focus on our challenges, but focus on our abilities! Say that again, "Focus on your abilities!" Bear Bryant said, "If you believe in yourself and have dedication and pride - and never quit, you WILL be a winner. The price of victory is high but so are the rewards."

**Aerobic-Surges:**

1) (Touch the floor and jump to the ceiling 120 times)
2) ________________________________________
3) ________________________________________
4) ________________________________________
5) ________________________________________

**Meals and Snacks:**

1. ________________________________________
2. ________________________________________
3. (Take Quick Salsa to work with chicken)
4. ________________________________________
5. ________________________________________

**Challenges:**

**Victories:**

## Day 29

**Tips:** Walt Disney once said, “All our dreams can come true – if we have the courage to pursue them.” He also said, “If you can dream, you can do it. Always remember that this whole thing was started by a mouse!” You’ve almost reached your 30-day victory and now write down your 3, 6, and 12 month victories that you Will See!

**Aerobic-Surges:**

1) (Calf Raises and Jumps)

2)

3)

4)

5)

**Meals and Snacks:**

1.

2.

3. (Take Salmon Salad to work; make other jealous!)

4.

5.

**Challenges:**

**Victories:**

**Day 30**

**Tips:** President John F. Kennedy said, "When written in Chinese, the word 'crisis' is composed of two characters—one represents danger, and the other represents opportunity."

**Aerobic-Surges:**

1) (Scissor Kicks with your Spouse not AT him!) ______
2) ____________________________________
3) ____________________________________
4) ____________________________________
5) ____________________________________

**Meals and Snacks:**

1. ____________________________________
2. ____________________________________
3. (Spiced green beans with crockpot chicken) ______
4. ____________________________________
5. ____________________________________

**Challenges:**

**Victories:**

**DO NOT just read through this and set your book aside! Start today with an Energy-surge.** "Never put off until, tomorrow, what you can perform TODAY!"
~ Benjamin Franklin

***Digest this:*** The first step to losing weight is to stop gaining weight! When in doubt, move it out and ***do another aerobic surge every time you think of it.*** Forecast your day and you success Will BE on your horizon!

**Cheers to your Victory!**

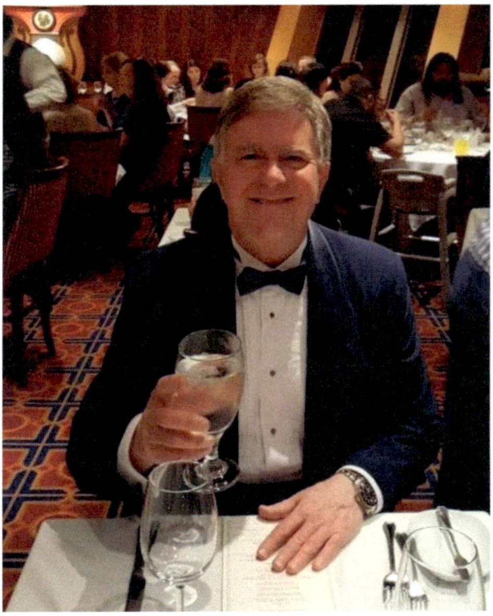

## KEY RESOURCES

**www.DocWillis.org**

www.WedMD.com

http://www.**Medscape**.com/

http://www.**cdc.go**v/nccdphp/dnpa/nutrition/pdf/**portion_size_research**.pdf

http://www.mayoclinic.com/**health/water**/NU00283

www.HealthyPeople.gov

http://www.LiveStrong.com

www.ChooseMyPlate.gov

http://www.lifescript.com/

**American Dietetic Association**

http://www.eatright.org

**US Department of Agriculture Center for Nutrition** http://www.usda.gov/cnpp

**USDA Dietary Guidelines**

http://www.nal.usda.gov/fnic/dga/index.html

**The Interactive Food Guide Pyramid**

http://www.nal.usda.gov:8001/py/pmap.htm

**Nutrition and Athletic Performance**

http://www.ms-se.com

**Supplement Information**

http://www.acsm.org/health+fitness/comments.htm

**NOTES:**

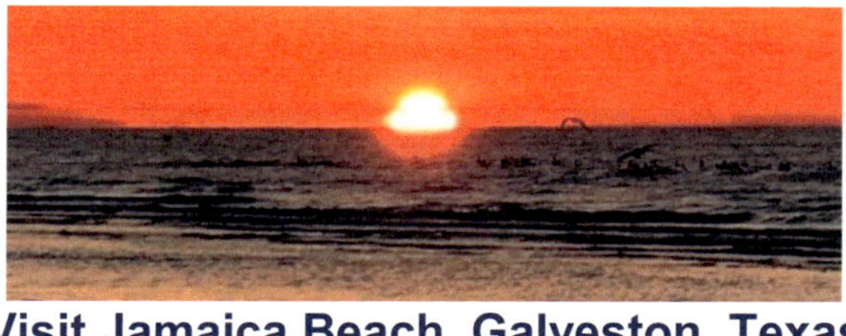

## KEY REFERENCES:

1) Willis FB, Shanmugam R, Curran, SA. **Food Allergen Eliminations and Combined Protocols for Obesity Reduction: a Preliminary Comparison Study**. *Food Science & Nutrition Research*. Nov. 2018;1:1

2) *Willis FB. RightSize Weight Loss*. (Evergreen Press, Mobile AL, USA, 2016.)

3) Willis, FB. *Effective Orthopedic Rehab, Seven Steps to Complete Recovery.* Trafford Publishing, Victoria Canada, 2003.

4) Willis FB, Smith FM, Willis AP. **Frequency of exercise for body fat loss: a controlled, cohort study**. *J Strength Cond Res.* 2009 Nov; 23(8):2377-80.

5) McKeith G. *You are what you eat*. (Plume Publishing, London Engkand, 2006)

6) Lewis JE, Woolger JM, Melillo A, et al. **Eliminating immunologically-reactive foods from the diet and its effect on body composition and quality of life in overweight persons.** J Obes Weig loss Ther. 2012; 2:112.

7) **CDC Obesity rates** (viewed August 2018) http://www.cdc.gov/obesity/data/adult.html

8) Chen J. **Making a Case for Food Sensitivity Testing**, *Huffington Post*

https://www.huffingtonpost.com/julie-chen-md/making-a-case-for-food-se_b_8387196.html (viewed August 2018)

9) Rivera R, Deutsch RD. *Your Hidden Food Allergies Are Making You Fat*. (2002) Three Rivers Press, NY, USA.

10) "**Food Allergy Basics: Facts and Statistics**," Food Allergy Research and Education, https://www.foodallergy.org/facts-and-stats

11) Alpay K, Ertaş M, Orhan EK, Üstay DK, Lieners C, Baykan B. **Diet restriction in migraine, based on IgG against foods: A clinical double-blind, randomized, cross-over trial.** *Cephalalgia* . 2010;30(7):829-837.

12) Kesman RL, Ebbert JO, Harris KI, Schroeder DR. **Portion control for the treatment of obesity in the primary care setting**. *BMC Res Notes.* 2011 Sep 9;4:346.

13) Torbahn G, Gellhaus I, Koch B, et al. **Reduction of Portion Size and Eating Rate Is Associated with BMI-SDS Reduction in Overweight and Obese Children and Adolescents: Results on Eating and Nutrition Behaviour from the Observational KgAS Study.** Obes Facts. 2017;10(5):503-516.

14) Iwao S, Mori K, Sato Y. **Effects of meal frequency on body composition during weight control in boxers**. *Scand J Med Sci Sports.* 1996 Oct;6(5):265-72.

15) Fisher G, Brown AW, Bohan Brown MM, et al. **High Intensity Interval- vs Moderate Intensity- Training for Improving Cardiometabolic Health in**

**Overweight or Obese Males: A Randomized Controlled Trial.** *PLoS One.* 2015 Oct 21;10(10).

16)Torbahn G, Gellhaus I, Koch B, et al. **Reduction** of **Portion Size** and **Eating Rate Is Associated with BMI-SDS Reduction in Overweight and Obese Children and Adolescents: Results on Eating and Nutrition Behaviour from the Observational KgAS Study.** *Obes Facts.* 2017;10(5):503-516.

17)Daley, AJ, Copeland, RJ, Wright, NP, Roalfe, A, and Wales, JK. **Exercise therapy as a treatment for psychopathologic conditions in obese and morbidly obese adolescents: a randomized, controlled trial.** *Pediatrics.* 2006 Nov;118(5):2126-34.

18)De Feo P. **Is high-intensity exercise better than moderate-intensity exercise for weight loss?** *Nutr Metab Cardiovasc Dis.* 2013 Nov;23(11):1037-42.

19)Grossman JA, Payne EK. **A randomized comparison study regarding the impact of short-duration, high-intensity exercise and traditional exercise on anthropometric and body composition measurement changes in post-menopausal women-A pilot study**. *Post Reprod Health.* 2016 Mar;22(1):14-9.

20)Sijie T, Hainai Y, Fengying Y, Jianxiong W. **High intensity interval exercise training in overweight young women.** *J Sports Med Phys Fitness.* 2012 Jun;52(3):255-62.

21)Poulsen SK, Due A, Jordy AB, et al. **Health effect of the New Nordic Diet in adults with increased waist**

**circumference: a 6-mo randomized controlled trial**. *Am J Clin Nutr.* 2014 Jan;99(1):35-45.

22)Palmer DJ, Huang RC, Craig JM, Prescott SL. **Nutritional influences on epigenetic programming: asthma, allergy, and obesity**. *Immunol Allergy Clin North Am.* 2014 Nov;34(4):825-37.

23) Fries WC. **The Natural Diet: Best Foods for Weight Loss** https://www.webmd.com/diet/features/the-natural-diet-best-foods-for-weight-loss#1 t (Viewed Nov 2017)

24)Hurtado-Barroso S, Tresserra-Rimbau A, Vallverdú-Queralt A, Lamuela-Raventós RM. **Organic food and the impact on human health**. *Crit Rev Food Sci Nutr.* 2017 Nov 30:1-11.

25)Pergola G, Foroni F, Mengotti P, Argiris G, Rumiati RI. **A neural signature of food semantics is associated with body-mass index**. *Biol Psychol.* 2017 Oct;129:282-292.

26)John Berardi The Metabolism Advantage, Rodale press, 2006

27)Willis FB, Curran S. A **Brief, Aerobic-surge Exercises for Effective Weight Loss: a Randomized, Controlled Trial.** (In-press: *International Medicine*)

28)Diliberti N, Bordi PL, Conklin MT, Roe LS, Rolls BJ. **Increased portion size leads to increased energy intake in a restaurant meal**. *Obes Res.* 2004 Mar;12(3):562-8.

29)Rolls BJ, Morris EL, Roe LS. **Portion size of food affects energy intake in normal-weight and overweight men and women**. *Am J Clin Nutr.* 2002 Dec;76(6):1207-13.

30)Foster TM, Sumpter CE, Temple W, Flevill A, Poling A. **Demand equations for qualitatively different foods under fixed-ratio schedules: a comparison of three data conversions**. *J Exp Anal Behav.* 2009 Nov;92(3):305-26.

31)Shin KO, Moritani T. **The combined effects of capsaicin, green tea extract and chicken essence tablets on human autonomic nervous system activity**. *J Nutr Sci Vitaminol* (Tokyo). 2007 Apr;53(2):145-52.

32)Dulloo AG, Seydoux J, Girardier L, Chantre P, Vandermander J. **Green tea and thermogenesis: interactions between catechin-polyphenols, caffeine and sympathetic activity**. *Int J Obes Relat Metab Disord.* 2000 Feb;24(2):252-8.

33)Cohen-Sharir Y, Kuperman Y, Apelblat D, den Hertog J, **Spiegel** I, Knobler H, Elson A. **Protein tyrosine phosphatase alpha inhibits hypothalamic leptin receptor signaling and regulates body weight in vivo**. *FASEB J.* 2019 Apr;33(4):5101-5111.

34)Copinschi G, Leproult R, Spiegel K. **The important role of sleep in metabolism.** *Front Horm Res.* 2014;42:59-72.

35)Bilcu M, Grumezescu AM, Oprea AE, Popescu RC, Mogoșanu GD, Hristu R, Stanciu GA, Mihailescu DF, Lazar V, Bezirtzoglou E, Chifiriuc MC. **Efficiency of**

**vanilla, patchouli and ylang ylang essential oils stabilized by iron oxide@C14 nanostructures against bacterial adherence and biofilms formed by Staphylococcus aureus and Klebsiella pneumoniae clinical strains**. *Molecules.* 2014 Nov 4;19(11):17943-56.

36)Momtazi-Borojeni AA, Esmaeili SA, Abdollahi E, Sahebkar A. A **Review on the Pharmacology and Toxicology of Steviol Glycosides Extracted from Stevia rebaudiana**. *Curr Pharm Des.* 2017;23(11):1616-1622.

37)Porter NT, Martens EC.**The Critical Roles of Polysaccharides in Gut Microbial Ecology and Physiology**. *Annu Rev Microbiol.* 2017 Sep 8;71:349-369.

38) PubMEd (seen Sept. 2019) https://www.ncbi.nlm.nih.gov/pmc/articles/PMC6315330/

39) Stanislavov R, Rohdewald P. **Improvement of erectile function by a combination of French maritime pine bark and roburins with aminoacids**. *Minerva Urol Nefrol.* 2015 Mar;67(1):27-32.

40) Ito TY, Polan ML, Whipple B, Trant AS. **The enhancement of female sexual function with ArginMax, a nutritional supplement, among women differing in menopausal status**. *J Sex Marital Ther.* 2006 Oct-Dec;32(5):369-78.

**Body Summation Score**

Physician's name____________________ date_____

Body Weight (kg)____ Height (m)____ BMI____

BMI= weight kg ÷ height$^2$ (meters)

For example 220 lbs. = 100kg, 70" = 1.78m

100kg ÷ (1.78)2 = 31.6 BMI is obese

Current Dress or Pant Size _____

**Girth Measurements** (use measuring tape)

Neck ____

Shoulders ____

Upper Arm ____

Chest ____

Waist ____ (widest girth)

Hips ____

Upper thigh ____ (widest girth)

Above knee ____ (2" above knee cap)

Calf ____

**Girth Total** ____

Contact us and we will help yuou find the testing center (BodPod or DEXA) to measure Body Fat.

**Total Body Fat** ____% x weight = ____ mass

Visceral Fat ____ Total Muscle mass ____

**Body Summation Score**

Physician's name____________________ date_____

Body Weight (kg)____ Height (m)____ BMI____

BMI= weight kg ÷ height$^2$ (meters)

For example 220 lbs. = 100kg, 70" = 1.78m

100kg ÷ (1.78)2 = 31.6 BMI is obese

Current Dress or Pant Size _____

**Girth Measurements** (use measuring tape)

Neck ____

Shoulders ____

Upper Arm ____

Chest ____

Waist ____ (widest girth)

Hips ____

Upper thigh ____ (widest girth)

Above knee ____ (2" above knee cap)

Calf ____

**Girth Total** ____

Contact us and we will help yuou find the testing center (BodPod or DEXA) to measure Body Fat.

**Total Body Fat** ____% x weight = ____ mass

Visceral Fat ____ Total Muscle mass ____

For Color Pictures of Recipes and the 2-minute

Aerobic-surge exercises go to

**www.DrBuckWillis.com**

**Please give us a 5-Star Review on Amazon and**

contact me if you need more help!

FBW@DocWillis.org

*Cheers, Doc ><>*

Made in the USA
Las Vegas, NV
03 November 2026

57424981R00143